PHYSIOLOGICAL PHARMACEUTICS
Biological Barriers to Drug Absorption

ELLIS HORWOOD SERIES IN PHARMACEUTICAL TECHNOLOGY

Editor: Professor M. H. RUBINSTEIN, School of Health Sciences, Liverpool Polytechnic

EXPERIMENTAL DRUG DESIGN: Pharmaceutical Applications
N. A. Armstrong & K. C. James
MICROBIAL QUALITY ASSURANCE IN PHARMACEUTICALS, COSMETICS AND TOILETRIES
Edited by S. Bloomfield *et al.*
DRUG DISCOVERY TECHNOLOGIES: An Eighties Perspective
C. Clark & W. H. Moos
PHARMACEUTICAL PRODUCTION FACILITIES: Design and Applications
G. Cole
PHARMACEUTICAL TABLET AND PELLET COATING
G. Cole
THE PHARMACY AND PHARMACOTHERAPY OF ASTHMA
Edited by P. F. D'Arcy & J. C. McElnay
PHARMACEUTICAL THERMAL ANALYSIS: Techniques and Applications
J. L. Ford and P. Timmins
PHYSICO-CHEMICAL PROPERTIES OF DRUGS: A Handbook for Pharmaceutical Scientists
P. Gould
HANDBOOK OF PHARMACOKINETICS: Toxicity Assessment of Chemicals
J. P. Labaune
TABLET MACHINE INSTRUMENTATION IN PHARMACEUTICS: Principles and Practice
P. Ridgway Watt
PHARMACEUTICAL CHEMISTRY, Volume 1 Drug Synthesis
H. J. Roth *et al.*
PHARMACEUTICAL CHEMISTRY, Volume 2 Drug Analysis*
H. J. Roth *et al.*
PHARMACEUTICAL TECHNOLOGY: Controlled Drug Release, Volume 1
Edited by M. H. Rubinstein
PHARMACEUTICAL TECHNOLOGY: Controlled Drug Release, Volume 2*
Edited by M. H. Rubinstein
PHARMACEUTICAL TECHNOLOGY: Tableting Technology, Volume 1
Edited by M. H. Rubinstein
PHARMACEUTICAL TECHNOLOGY: Tableting Technology, Volume 2*
Edited by M. H. Rubinstein
PHARMACEUTICAL TECHNOLOGY: Drug Stability
Edited by M. H. Rubinstein
PHARMACEUTICAL TECHNOLOGY: Drug Targeting*
Edited by M. H. Rubinstein
UNDERSTANDING BACTERIAL RESISTANCE*
D. A. Russell and I. Chopra
UNDERSTANDING CELL TOXICOLOGY
R. Stenberg, *et al.*
RADIOPHARMACEUTICALS USING RADIOACTIVE COMPOUNDS IN PHARMACEUTICS AND MEDICINE
Edited by A. Theobald
PHARMACEUTICAL PREFORMULATION: The Physicochemical Properties of Drug Substances
J. I. Wells
DRUG DELIVERY AND THE GASTROINTESTINAL TRACT
C. Wilson
PHYSIOLOGICAL PHARMACEUTICS: Biological Barriers to Drug Absorption
C. G. Wilson & N. Washington

* *In preparation*

PHYSIOLOGICAL PHARMACEUTICS
Biological Barriers to Drug Absorption

CLIVE G. WILSON B.Sc., Ph.D.

NEENA WASHINGTON B.Sc., Ph.D.

both of Department of Physiology and Pharmacology
Queen's Medical Centre, Nottingham

ELLIS HORWOOD LIMITED
Publishers · Chichester

Halsted Press: a division of
JOHN WILEY & SONS
New York · Chichester · Brisbane · Toronto

First published in 1989 by
ELLIS HORWOOD LIMITED
Market Cross House, Cooper Street,
Chichester, West Sussex, PO19 1EB, England
The publisher's colophon is reproduced from James Gillison's drawing of the ancient Market Cross, Chichester.

Distributors:

Australia and New Zealand:
JACARANDA WILEY LIMITED
GPO Box 859, Brisbane, Queensland 4001, Australia

Canada:
JOHN WILEY & SONS CANADA LIMITED
22 Worcester Road, Rexdale, Ontario, Canada

Europe and Africa:
JOHN WILEY & SONS LIMITED
Baffins Lane, Chichester, West Sussex, England

North and South America and the rest of the world:
Halsted Press: a division of
JOHN WILEY & SONS
605 Third Avenue, New York, NY 10158, USA

South-East Asia
JOHN WILEY & SONS (SEA) PTE LIMITED
37 Jalan Pemimpin # 05–04
Block B, Union Industrial Building, Singapore 2057

Indian Subcontinent
WILEY EASTERN LIMITED
4835/24 Ansari Road
Daryaganj, New Delhi 110002, India

© 1989 C.G. Wilson and N. Washington/Ellis Horwood Limited

British Library Cataloguing in Publication Data
Wilson, Clive George
Physiological pharmaceutics.
1. Man. Drugs. Absorption
I. Title II. Washington, Neena
615'.7

Library of Congress Card no. 89–19884

ISBN 0–7458–0543–4 (Ellis Horwood Limited)
ISBN 0–470–21545–3 (Halsted Press)

Printed in Great Britain by The Camelot Press, Southampton

Table of contents

Preface

This book originated from the notes produced for the lecture course "Physiological Constraints in Oral Drug Delivery", a part of the European Continuing Education College scheme. The notes had to include all of the material used for the three-day lecture course. At the end of preparing this, we foolishly believed that we were three-quarters of the way to producing a book, but we were wrong! Two years later we finally made it, with the help of our colleagues, Jane Greaves, Clive Washington, Karen Steed and Elaine Blackshaw, who contributed to the book, gave us moral support and tolerated us in our worst moments!

The book, as with the lecture course from which it originated, attempts to bridge the gaps between the classical courses of Pharmacy and Biological Sciences. We have not emphasised the mathematical aspects of the physical chemistry, but tried to put it into the context of the biological environment in which the drugs and dosage forms are expected to perform.

New sophisticated delivery systems for existing drugs have been introduced over the last 20 years due to the high cost of development of new entities. In order for innovative pharmaceutics to be successful *in vivo*, the drugs and dosage forms have to be designed to overcome the body's barrier mechanisms which have specifically evolved to exclude foreign material, with the further complication of concomitant physiological processes which affect factors such as availablility of fluid for dissolution, enzymes, pH etc.

The majority of drugs are administered via the oral route. The gastrointestinal tract is often described as a tube linking mouth to anus, however not only does the environment within the lumen and the capacity for drug absorption vary drastically throughout its length, but the presence or absence of food affects both motility and secretion. The overall scenario is complex and hence five chapters of the book have been devoted to this area. Ophthalmic, nasal and pulmonary routes for drug delivery are also main research areas of our group and we have used the technique of gamma scintigraphy to investigate drug delivery, deposition and residence in these organs. The production of the chapter on transdermal drug delivery required the invaluable help of our colleague, Dr Clive Washington. Due to the restraints of time and length of the text, the other routes of administration such as subcutaneous, intramuscular and vaginal were not covered in this book. We plan to cover these subjects in a later text when we have summoned up sufficient energy and courage to take on such a large task!

Nottingham 1989   *Neena Washington*
                                                    Clive Wilson

1

Overview of Epithelial Barriers and Drug Transport

Clive Wilson, Clive Washington* and Neena Washington
*Department of Pharmaceutical Sciences, Nottingham University,
University Park, Nottingham, NG7 2RD.

Most systemically or locally acting drugs have to pass through epithelial cell layers to reach the target tissue in order to produce a pharmacological action. Differences in the cell types, the manner in which they are joined together to form layers and the microenvironment produced by cell secretions, results in a diversity of character-istics of epithelial barrier.

Epithelial barriers delineate the outer margins of organs, possessing structural, secretory and absorptive elements in a heterogeneous organisation. In common with other cell types, provision must be made for the supply and retention of substrates from extracellular sources and the secretion of waste products which would otherwise accumulate in toxic amounts. The outer membrane of the cell must therefore allow penetration of some substances and not others, i.e. it must be selectively permeable. This is one of the most important features of the cell boundary or plasma membrane.

STRUCTURE OF THE PLASMA MEMBRANE

Early researchers recognised that hydrophobic materials entered cells easily and proposed that an oily or 'lipoidal' barrier was present at the cell surface. Gorter and Grendel (1925) estimated the thickness of this layer by extracting the oily membrane from erythrocytes with acetone and spreading it as a monomolecular film in a trough. By measuring the film area and calculating the surface area of the original red cells, they concluded that exactly two layers of molecules were present at the interface, and proposed a lipid bilayer as the major cell membrane element. We now know that their experiment was subject to a considerable number of errors (Bar *et al.,* 1966), but fortunately these cancelled out in the final analysis and hence they obtained the correct answer by the wrong route! Electron micrographs indicated a double layered lipid membrane with bands approximately 3 nm in width and an overall thickness of between 8 to 12 nm.

The chemical nature of the lipids was gradually elucidated in the following decades, particularly after the introduction of chromatography; we now know that there are several hundred lipoidal molecules, including phospholipids, sphingolipids, and sterols. The amphipathic phospholipids are aligned to form a bilayer with the hydrophilic head groups on the outer surface and the hydrophobic fatty acid chains in the interior. The outer cell surface also frequently possesses a diffuse layer of mucopolysaccharide attached as glycolipids. Later experiments demonstrated that a variable fraction of many membranes was composed of proteins; several structures were proposed to account for this, but the most useful is the fluid mosaic model proposed by Singer and Nicholson (1972) (Figure 1.1). The surfaces of the membrane are composed of tightly packed phospholipids interspersed with proteins. The proteins were originally thought to float in a sea of lipid, leading to a rather ill-defined mixed membrane. However, studies during the last decade have demonstrated that the membrane is a highly organised structure; proteins in specific conformations act as structural elements, transport nutrients, and sample the cell environment. The bilayer is not a lipid 'sea' but a carefully designed liquid crystal whose composition is controlled by the cell to achieve a specific degree of fluidity and an optimum environment for the processes which occur within it.

Fluidity of the membrane allows processes such as pinocytosis to occur. When alveolar macrophages or polymorphonuclear leucocytes are allowed to ingest inert latex particles or oil droplets, more than half of the original plasma membrane may

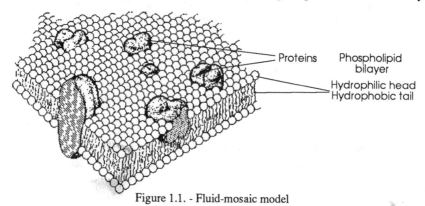

Figure 1.1. - Fluid-mosaic model

be taken up into the cell (Quinn, 1976). Certain components such as transport proteins are left on the cell surface, while others are removed roughly in proportion to the amount of membrane internalised. The fluid mosaic model gives the impression of lateral mobility of the proteins within the lipid environment, although lectin binding sites have been shown to be anchored firmly into the membrane and are not free to move laterally (Bittinger and Schnebli, 1974). Some cells, such as those of the intestinal mucosa, show stable differentiation of the plasma membrane to form protrusions called microvilli. These normally occur on the luminal side of epithelia to increase adsorptive area and are known as brush borders due to their appearance in electronmicrographs.

The interior of the membrane is more loosely ordered since the embedded proteins cause discontinuities in the structure. Some of the proteins protrude through the surface and make contact with the aqueous phases on both sides of the membrane. These subunits form components of the specialised transport systems such as the membrane ATPases and those for polar compounds including glucose and sodium.

Nearly all biological membranes possess a characteristic spectrum of enzyme activity. Membrane bound enzymes are intercalated to form an integral part of the structure and cannot be removed by washing. Other membrane proteins are present which are not enzymes, and their function may be structural, exerting a limited organisational effect on membrane components in their vicinity. Finally, membranes may provide an environment for receptors, both for chemical stimuli and for sensory factors such as light.

EPITHELIA
With a few exceptions, all internal and external body surfaces are covered with epithelium. There are several epithelial cell types (Figure 1.2):
a) Simple squamous epithelium which forms a thin layer. This type of epithelium lines most of the blood vessels.
b) Simple columnar epithelium. A single layer of columnar cells is found in areas such as the stomach and small intestine.
c) Stratified epithelial membranes. These membranes are several cells thick and are found in areas which have to withstand large amounts of wear and tear, for example the inside of the mouth and oesophagus.

Epithelial cells are said to be polarised due to the asymmetric distribution of transport proteins on their opposite plasma membranes. This causes the transport activity of the apex of the cell to be different to that of the basolateral membrane. For example sodium has to cross two types of barrier to enter the blood from the lumen. At the apex of the cell, sodium is actively transported into the cell by a carrier-mediated mechanism along a concentration gradient. At the base of the cell sodium is extruded by an active carrier mechanism against an electrochemical potential.

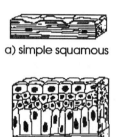

a) simple squamous

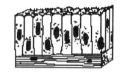

b) simple columnar

c) transitional

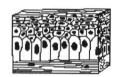

d) stratified squamous
(non-keratinised)

Figure 1.2. - Different epithelial cell types

CELL JUNCTIONS

The epithelium is not a continuous layer and divisions between the cells are seen by light microscopy. There are three types of cell junctions (Figure 1.3):
a) tight junctions or *zonulae occludens*
b) gap junctions
c) desmosomes or *zonulae adherens*.

Tight Junctions

Tight junctions are formed when specific proteins in two interacting plasma membranes make direct contact across the intercellular space (Figure 1.4). These can be visualized as linear strands of intermembrane proteins. A belt-like structure composed of many protein strands completely encircles each cell in the sheet, attaching it to its neighbours. At a tight junction, the interacting plasma membranes are so closely apposed that there is no intercellular space and the membranes are within 2Å of each other. As these junctions can be disrupted either by treatment with proteolytic enzymes or by agents that chelate Ca^{2+} or Mg^{2+}, both the proteins and divalent cations are required for maintaining their integrity. Beneath the tight junction, the adjacent cells are relatively free to widen their separating spaces depending on different physiological conditions. (Esposito, 1984). The structure has been likened to "a six-pack of beer extended indefinitely in 2 dimensions" (Diamond, 1977).

Tight junctions play a crucial part in maintaining the selective barrier function of cell sheets. For example, the epithelial cells lining the small intestine must keep most of the gut contents in the lumen; simultaneously, the cells must pump selected nutrients across the cell sheet into the extracellular fluid on the other side, from which they are absorbed into the blood.

Tight junctions make transport possible in two different ways:
(i) they act as diffusion barriers within the lipid bilayer of the plasma membrane, thus, they prevent the transport proteins

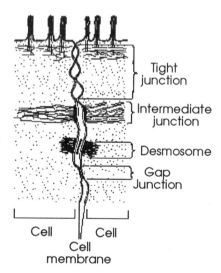

Tight junction

Intermediate junction

Desmosome

Gap Junction

Cell   Cell

Cell membrane

Figure 1.3. - Different types of cell junctions

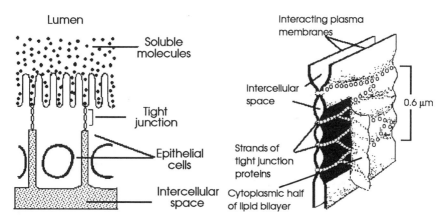

Figure 1.4. - Tight junctions hold cells together at their apical end (left) and an enlargement (right)

in the apical membrane from diffusing into the basolateral membrane, and vice versa.

(ii) they seal neighbouring cells together to create a continuous sheet of cells between which even small molecules are unable to pass.

Gap Junctions

The commonest type of cell junction is the gap junction, which is widely distributed in tissues of all animals (Figure 1.3). They are characterized by regions in which the cell membranes are separated by a gap 2 to 3 nm wide. The 'gap' is crossed by cytoplasmic filaments which allow intracellular cytoplasm to transfer between cells. Molecules up to 1200 Daltons can pass freely between the cells but larger molecules cannot, suggesting a functioning pore size for the connecting channels of about 1.5 nm. This pore size implies that coupled cells share a variety of small molecules (such as inorganic ions, sugars, amino acids, nucleotides and vitamins) but do not share their macromolecules (proteins, nucleic acids and polysaccharides). Cyclic AMP is a molecule which is known to pass through gap junctions, which implies that hormonal stimulation in just one or a few epithelial cells will initiate a metabolic response in many cells. Gap junctions will close in the presence of high concentrations of Ca^{2+} ions.

Desmosomes

Desmosomes are widely distributed in tissues, where they enable groups of cells to function as structural units. They are most abundant in tissues that are subject to severe mechanical stress, such as cardiac muscle, skin epithelium and the neck of the uterus, suggesting that they are important for holding cells together. Desmosomes can be divided into three different types: spot desmosomes, belt desmosomes and hemidesmosomes, all three of which are present in most epithelial cells.

Belt desmosomes form a continuous band around each of the interacting cells in an epithelial sheet, near the cell's apical end. The bands in adjacent cells are directly apposed and are separated by a poorly characterized filamentous material (in the intercellular space) that presumably holds the interacting membranes together. Within each cell, contractile bundles of actin filaments run along the belts just under the plasma membrane. These filament bundles probably mediate one of the most fundamental processes in animal morphogenesis - the folding of epithelial cell sheets into tubes.

Spot desmosomes act like rivets to hold epithelial cells together at button-like points of contact. They also serve as anchoring sites for keratin filaments which extend from one side of the cell to the other across the cell interior, forming a structural framework for the cytoplasm. Since other filaments extend from cell to cell at spot desmosomes, the keratin filament networks inside adjacent cells are connected indirectly through these junctions to form a continuous network of fibres across the entire epithelial sheet.

Hemidesmosomes or half-desmosomes resemble spot desmosomes, but instead of joining adjacent epithelial cell membranes together, they join the basal surface of epithelial cells to the underlying basal lamina. Together spot desmosomes and hemidesmosomes act as rivets that distribute any shearing force through the epithelial sheet and its underlying connective tissue.

PASSAGE OF MOLECULES INTO THE BODY
Inter and Intracellular Routes of Absorption
The exchange of substances between individual cells and the interstitial fluid occurs at the plasma membrane. In the body specialised epithelial surfaces constitute the interface where the exchange of substances between the body and its environment occurs. These tissues, which include intestinal mucosa, lung alveoli, renal tubules and skin, consist of one or more layers of cells, but ultimately it is the particular properties of the membrane which regulate the passage of substances into the body.

Molecules can pass from the lumen into the bloodstream via two routes:
a) transcellularly, in which the molecules are transported into and through epithelial cells and transferred into the bloodstream. This can occur either as a result of passive transport, active transport or membrane invagination.
b) intercellularly, in which molecules pass directly into the bloodstream via the junctions between the epithelial cells.

The Transcellular Route
Passage though the cells of the absorbing epithelium involves permeation across the brush border, the intracellular space and the basolateral membrane. Small molecules such as water and small hydrophobic solutes pass into the epithelial cells by passive transport. This is simply due to diffusion down a concentration gradient. The rate of passive transport depends on the solubility of the molecule in the lipid bilayer and is greater for molecules with large oil-water partition coefficients.

pH-partition hypothesis

Drug molecules dissolved in the aqueous environment are predominantly weakly ionisable species containing groups such as amine, carboxyl, phenol, etc. These materials are absorbed across plasma membranes in their unionised forms, since these are non-polar; the ionised forms of the drug cannot pass through the membrane due to its hydrophobic character. Consequently the pH of the microenvironment is critical in determining the absorption across the membrane. Thus, for example, an acidic drug is absorbed from acidic solution since it will be in its unionised protonated form. This is the basis of the pH-partition hypothesis, stressed in most classical texts of pharmacology, which estimate the absorption of drug on the basis of the relative degrees of ionisation in the lumen and the blood.

The pH-partition hypothesis provides an indication of drug absorption, but suffers from many shortcomings. The most notable of these can be seen in the widely quoted example of the absorption of an acidic drug from the stomach, in which the acidic drug is in its unionised state at pH 2 (the stomach) and so passes across the membrane. In the blood (at pH 7.4) the drug is ionised, and so cannot pass back across the membrane. This effect is referred to as ion-trapping. The conclusion is that pH and ionisation are highly important. This represents not only the most extreme example available of pH gradient *in vivo*, but it also should be remembered that drug absorption from the stomach is extremely small and most absorption takes place in the small intestine which is normally close to pH 7. Here the ionisation of the drug in the lumen is similar to that in the blood and little ion-trapping can occur. Gastric contents delivered into the duodenum make the first few centimetres acidic, until the chyme has been neutralised by bicarbonate, but transit through this region is extremely rapid and so no significant absorption can occur.

The biggest failing of this hypothesis is to attempt to calculate absorption from equilibrium drug distributions, when in practise the absorbed drug is swept away by the circulation. Absorption is a dynamic process involving dissolution, ionization, partition and blood flow and consequently correlation with experiment is poor.

Facilitated and carrier-mediated diffusion

Ions will not pass through the lipid bilayer but may be transported by membrane proteins providing hydrophilic transport channels. As this process also is driven by the concentration gradient it is referred to as facilitated diffusion or carrier-mediated diffusion. The major characteristic of this process is that it is saturable when the transport protein is fully utilised, i.e. it follows Michaelis-Menten kinetics. Glucose and other medium-sized molecules can be transported in this manner. The term facilitated diffusion is also often applied to the case in which blood flow or protein binding removes diffused drug and hence maintains a concentration gradient.

Molecules which travel against a concentration gradient must be absorbed by active transport since energy is required for this process. The best-studied systems of this type are the ATPase transport proteins which are particularly important in maintaining concentration gradients of small ions in cells, such as nerve cells. These proteins use the energy of hydrolysis of ATP to exchange different ions on opposite sides of the membrane. Thus, for example, the $H^+K^+ATPase$ found in the gastric parietal cells pumps hydrogen ions into the gastric lumen in exchange for potassium ions; this exchange process ensures electrical neutrality.

Absorption of many molecules occurs by co-transport, a variety of active transport in which the absorption into the cell against the concentration gradient is linked to the secretion of a cellular ion such as sodium down its concentration gradient. This process is important for the absorption of glucose and amino acids in the small intestine.

All the above mechanisms absorb only small molecules. There is evidence that larger molecules can be absorbed with low efficiency due to endocytosis. This may be divided into pinocytosis and phagocytosis. Pinocytosis is a process in which the cell membrane produces a deep infolding which is eventually detached as an intracellular vesicle. Subsequently the membrane of this vesicle is removed and the contents of the vesicle emptied into the cytosol. Pinocytosis is differentiated from phagocytosis, since pinocytosis involves the capture of extracellular liquid and is a property of most nucleated animal cells, whereas phagocytosis is a phenomenon associated with a few specialised cell types such as macrophages and neutrophils. Pinocytosis appears to be more substrate specific than the phagocytosis.

Little is known about the possible role of pinocytosis in the intestinal absorption of drugs and toxic substances. Pinocytosis may be involved in the absorption of vitamin B12. Large molecules such as botulinus toxin (900,000 Daltons) are examples which are quoted in favour of pinocytotic activity. Absorption of oral vaccines and polypeptides may also involve endocytosis.

Specific Transcellular Transport Mechanisms for Drugs
Although the absorption of most drugs can be explained by passive diffusion, some compounds have specific transport mechanisms. An example is the absorption in the intestine of some penicillin derivatives, e.g. cyclacillin (1 aminocyclohexyl-penicillin) (Csáky, 1984). This process is saturable, proceeds against an unfavorable concentration gradient and shows temperature dependence. Transport of amoxycillin is also carrier mediated but it is not an active process. Since these materials are xenobiotics, the transport mechanism is probably one which serves some other function in the body. The two penicillins probably share the same carrier since they are mutually competitive. Digitalis and other cardioselective glycosides also demonstrate a behaviour not compatible with simple partition theory which suggests carrier-mediated transport.

The Intercellular Route
Between cells epithelial brush borders come into close contact and under the electron microscope it appears as if the membrane is fused. However, functionally the tight junctions are not sealed but are permeable to water, electrolytes and other charged or uncharged molecules up to a certain size. The size of the "pore" varies

along the length of the gastrointestinal tract and can be calculated from recoveries of polyethylene glycols of various molecular weights (Chadwick *et al.*, 1977a,b). Intercellular transport may be important for oligosaccharides and small peptides, which is an area of considerable current interest.

There is a special mode of permeation across the intestinal wall in which the cell membranes are not involved. Intestinal cells are continuously produced in the crypts of Lieberkühn and migrate towards the tip of the villus. During digestion the cells are sloughed off leaving a temporary gap at the cell apex and through this gap large particles can slip into the circulation. This has been termed "persorption". The observation that large objects such as starch grains can be found in the blood after a meal of potatoes or corn is often

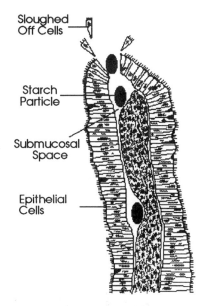

Figure 1.5. - Entrance of large particles into the submucosal space through the gap left by sloughed off cells (persorption)

quoted as the *prima facie* evidence of persorption or phagocytosis (Figure 1.5). Volkheimer and coworkers (1969) hypothesised that a "kneading" action of the villus on the luminal contents allowed particles of up to 100 μm diameter to enter the lamina propria of the intestinal mucosa near the apex of the villus. Metallic iron particles of up to 52 μm were identified in both portal venous blood and thoracic duct lymph of dogs after the animals were fed 200 g of iron powder suspended in milk and cream. Large foreign particles should be expected to enter intestinal lymph vessels in preference to mucosal blood vessels and it is remarkable that such large particles should appear at all in portal venous blood. It is possible that potentially harmful materials such as asbestos fibre can be absorbed in this way.

MUCUS

The majority of the epithelia discussed in this book are covered by a layer of mucus. The primary component of mucus is a large polysaccharide called mucin built up in subunits of 500,000 Daltons or larger. It consists of a protein backbone approximately 800 amino acids long, rich in serine, proline and threonine. Most of the hydroxy residues are linked to oligosaccharide side chains which serve to stiffen the backbone. The oligosaccharide chains are generally up to 18 residues in length and are composed of N-acetylgalactosamine, N-acetylglucosamine, galactose, fucose or N-acetylneuraminic acid.

Mucus serves as a lubricant and a protective layer. Its most important property is its viscoelasticity, which enables it to act as mechanical barrier and yet can flow under the influence of peristalsis. Mucus can exist in thicknesses of up to 600 μm before it begins to flow under it's own weight.

Mucus is 95% water and so makes intimate contact with hydrophilic surfaces. Small particles less than 600 μm may be buried in the surface and held securely due the stickiness of the mucus, but since the mucus is continually secreted the particles move further away from the mucosa and are ultimately sloughed off. Small molecules pass easily through mucus due to its high water content; larger molecules diffuse more slowly and remain in contact for longer periods. The concept of mucoadhesion is to use large molecules adhering to the mucus layer to bring drugs or delivery devices into close contact with the epithelium; however, mucus turnover can be rapid and there seems little point in attaching a drug to a surface which is to be sloughed off in a short time.

CONCLUSIONS
The absorption of drugs, although dependent on the site of absorption, is often controlled by the same set of barriers. These are mucus, hydrophobic membranes, transport processes and cell junctions. In the following chapters we will see how these barriers manifest themselves in different organs according to the form and function of the tissue involved.

REFERENCES
Bar R.S., Deamer D.W. and Cornwell D.G. (1966) Surface area of human erythrocyte lipids: reinvestigation of experiments on plasma membrane. *Science* **153** 1010-1012.

Bittinger H. and Schnebli H.P. (1974) Binding of concanavalin A and ricin to synaptic junctions of rat brain. *Nature* (Lond.) **249** 370-371.

Chadwick V.S., Phillips S.F. and Hofmann A.F. (1977a) Measurements of intestinal permeability using low molecular weight polyethylene glycols (PEG 400). 1. Chemical analysis and biological properties of PEG 400. *Gastroenterology* **73** 241-246.

Chadwick V.S., Phillips S.F. and Hofmann A.F. (1977b) Measurements of intestinal permeability using low molecular weight polyethylene glycols (PEG 400). 2. Application to normal and abnormal permeability states in man and animals. *Gastroenterology* **73** 247-251.

Csáky T.Z. (1984) Intestinal permeation and permeability: an overview. in *Pharmacology of Intestinal Permeation* Vol 1 ed. Csáky T.Z. Springer Verlag, Berlin pp 51-59.

Diamond J.M. (1977) The epithelial junction : bridge, gate and fence. *Physiologist* **20** 10-18.

Esposito G. (1984) Polarity of intestinal epithelial cells: permeability of the brush border and basolateral membranes. in *Pharmacology of Intestinal Permeation* Vol. 1 ed. Csáky T.Z. Springer Verlag, Berlin pp 283-308.

Gorter E. and Grendel F. (1925) Bimolecular layers of lipoids on chromatocytes of blood. *J. Exp. Med.* **41** 439-443.

Quinn P.J. (1976) The molecular biology of cell membranes. Macmillan Press, London.

Singer S.J. and Nicolson G.L. (1972) The fluid mosaic model of the structure of cell membranes. *Science* New York **175** 720-731.

Volkheimer G., Schulz F.H., Lindenau A. and Beitz U. (1969) Persorption of metallic iron particles. *Gut* **10** 32-33.

2

Drug Delivery to the Oral Cavity

The oral cavity is the point of entry for most drug formulations and usually their contact with the oral mucosa is brief. Venous return from the mouth enters the systemic circulation through the jugular vein and not the hepatic portal system. For this reason, first-pass metabolism is avoided and so there is much interest in optimising drug absorption from the oral epithelia. The nature, and hence the barrier properties, of the epithelial surface differs in the four major regions of potential drug absorption: palatal, buccal, sublingual and gingival (Figure 2.1).

ANATOMY AND PHYSIOLOGY OF THE ORAL CAVITY
The oral cavity is divided into two regions: (a) the outer oral vestibule, which is bounded by the cheeks and lips, and (b) the interior oral vestibule, which is bounded by the maxillary and mandibular arches, but the oral cavity proper is situated

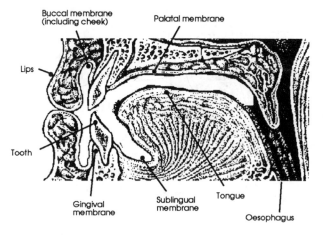

Figure 2.1. - Features of the buccal cavity illustrating changes in the epithelial lining

between the dental arches. At the back of the oral cavity are large collections of lymphoid tissue forming the tonsils; small lymphoid nodules may occur in the mucosa of the soft palate. This tissue plays an important role in combating infection.

Organisation of the Oral Mucosa
The oral mucosa is moist, relatively smooth and pink and there are several types, as shown in Figure 2.2.

The oral mucosa (Figure 2.3) is divided into
a) the oral epithelium
b) the basement membrane, which connects the epithelium to the connective tissue

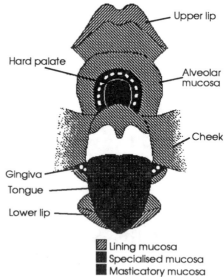

Figure 2.2. - The mucosa of the buccal cavity

c) the lamina propria, which is underlying connective tissue
d) an area which contains loose fatty or glandular connective tissue and major blood vessels and nerves. It is often referred to as the muco-periostium.
These tissues are laid over a layer of muscle or bone.

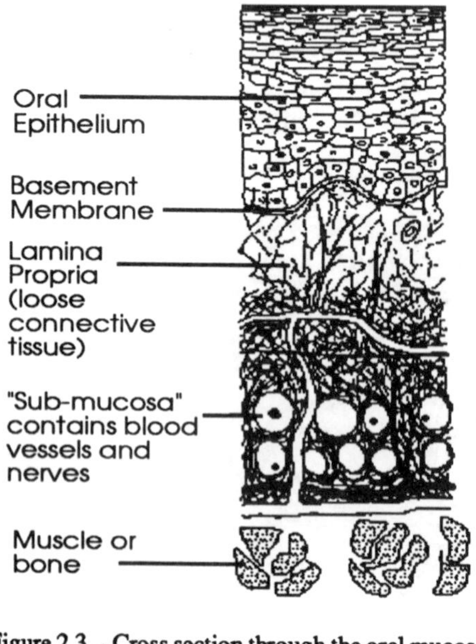

Oral Epithelium

Basement Membrane

Lamina Propria (loose connective tissue)

"Sub-mucosa" contains blood vessels and nerves

Muscle or bone

The epithelial lining of the oral mucosa is composed of squamous cells with a characteristic layered structure formed by the process of cell maturation. The composition of this layer varies according to the tissue functions; the hard palate and tongue, for example, are composed of keratinised epithelium whilst the lining of the cheek is distensible and non-keratinised. The thickness of the epithelium also varies in the buccal cavity (Table 2.1).

Sebaceous glands are found in the mucosa of 60 to 75% of adults and are seen as pale yellow spots in the upper lip and buccal mucosa. The openings of minor salivary glands are evident in many areas. In general, the oral mucosa has a more

Figure 2.3. - Cross section through the oral mucosa

Table 2.1. - Different types and thickness of epithelia in the buccal cavity
(from Veillard, 1987)

Tissue	Location	Thickness μm	Keratinisation	Polarity of lipids
Buccal	Cheek Upper and lower lip	500-600	No	Polar.
Sublingual	Frenulum Floor of mouth	100-200	No	Polar
Gingival	Gums	200	Yes	Non-polar
Palatal	Roof of mouth	250	Yes	Non-polar

concentrated network of vessels than is present in the skin. Almost all venous return from the oral mucosa enters the internal jugular vein. Lymphatic capillaries are also present in the lamina propria and arise as "blind" beginnings in the papillae.

Functions of the Oral Mucosa
The oral mucosa has similarities to both skin and intestinal mucosa. It has a protective role during the process of mastication, which exposes the mucosa to compression and shear forces. Areas such as the hard palate and attached gingiva have a horny surface to resist abrasion and are tightly bound to the underlying bone to resist shear forces. The cheek mucosae, on the other hand, are elastic to allow for distension.

The oral cavity contains the greatest variety of micro-organisms present within the human body. The entry into the body of these organisms and any potential toxic product is limited by the oral epithelium, which is not, as is often suggested, a highly permeable membrane.

The oral mucosa responds to the senses of pain, touch, and temperature in addition to its unique sense of taste. There are some protective mechanisms which respond to sensory input from the mouth, such as the initiation of swallowing, gagging and retching.

In some animals the oral mucosa is used to aid thermoregulation, for example panting in the dog. The human skin possesses sweat glands and a more highly controlled peripheral vasculature, so this role is thought to be minimal, although in sleep, dehydration results from prolonged breathing through the mouth.

Salivary Secretion
The major salivary glands are the parotid, submandibular (submaxillary) and sublingual gland (Figure 2.4). They are situated some way from the from the oral cavity, but open into it by a long duct. Minor salivary glands are situated in or immediately below the oral mucosa. The parotid and submaxillary glands produce

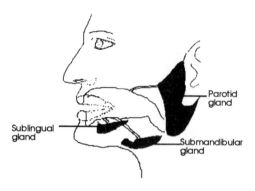

Figure 2.4. - The salivary glands

watery secretion, while the buccal and sublingual glands produce mainly viscous saliva.

Humans can produce up to 1 litre of saliva per day. The resting flow of saliva is 0.5 ml min⁻¹, which can be increased to more than 7 ml min⁻¹ upon maximal stimulation of the parasympathetic system, which exerts the major control over salivary secretion. Saliva is viscous, colourless and opalescent, hypotonic compared to plasma (between 110 and 220 milliosmoles per litre), with a specific gravity of about 1.003. The pH varies between 6.2 to 7.4 (low to high rates of flow), but the action of bacteria on sugar can reduce the pH to between 3 and 4 around the teeth. The composition of saliva depends upon the rate at which the different cell types contribute to the final secretion. The two types of secretion are mucous secretion, which is thick due to a glycoprotein called mucin, and watery secretion which contains salivary amylase. The major ions are Na^+, K^+, Cl^- and HCO_3^-. In the ducts of the salivary glands, sodium and chloride are reabsorbed, but potassium and bicarbonate are secreted (Figure 2.5) and hence the electrolyte balance is altered depending upon the rate of flow of saliva.

Enzymes detectable in saliva include an α-amylase, ptyalin, which begins to hydrolyse polysaccharides such as glycogen and starch to smaller saccharides. The enzyme has an optimum pH of 6.9, but is stable within the range 4 to 11 and hence it will continue to act until the food is acidified by gastric acid. The time of contact in the mouth is too short for digestion to occur but the enzyme may prevent accumulation of starchy material in the gaps between teeth. A lingual lipase is also present which hydrolyses triglycerides. It is extremely hydrophobic and its digestive action continues in the stomach.

There is potentially a high concentration of pathogenic bacteria present in the mouth which can easily destroy tissues and produce dental caries. The flow of saliva helps to wash the bacteria and the food particles, which act as their nutrient, into the acidic environment of the stomach where they are digested. Saliva also contains thiocyanate, protein antibodies and lysozyme which destroy the

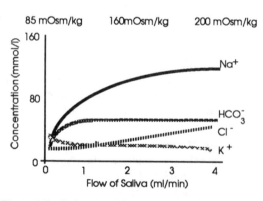

Figure 2.5. - Influence of flow on composition of saliva

bacteria. In the absence of saliva, oral ulcerations occur and dental caries becomes extremely prevalent. This condition, xerostomia, can be treated with artificial saliva formulations, which are based on materials such as hydroxypropylmethyl-cellulose and more recently, pig gastric mucin.

Saliva can be detected in the oral cavity soon after birth. Saliva secretion increases up to the age of 3 to 5 years, but then sharply declines, reaching a steady state by the age of 8 years. In adult females, the flow rate of saliva is somewhat lower than in males (Shannon and Prigmore, 1958).

ABSORPTION OF DRUGS ACROSS THE ORAL MUCOSA

The buccal cavity, like the entire alimentary canal, behaves as a lipoidal barrier to the passage of drugs. Active transport, pinocytosis, and passage through aqueous pores play only insignificant roles in moving drugs across the oral mucosa, although as discussed later, movement through the dentogingival margin may be important.

Absorption of drugs through the buccal mucosa was first described by Sobrero in 1847 who noted systemic effects produced by nitroglycerin after administration to the oral mucosa. The lingual route of administration became established in clinical practice in 1897 when William Murrell introduced nitroglycerin drops for the treatment of angina pectoris. Subsequently, nitroglycerin was formulated in tablets for sublingual use and was renamed glyceryl trinitrate.

The blood supply from the buccal mucosa and anal sphincter, unlike the remainder of the gastrointestinal tract, does not drain into the hepatic portal vein, since these peripheral areas are not specialised for the absorption of nutrients. Drugs which are absorbed through the oral mucosa thus enter the systemic circulation directly, avoiding passage through the liver where they might otherwise be metabolized; however, drug which is swallowed in the saliva does not avoid first pass metabo-lism, nor does it avoid degradation by digestive juices. The oral cavity is rich in blood vessels and lymphatics, so a rapid onset of action and high blood levels of drug are obtained quickly. In many cases buccal dose forms can have as high a bioavailability as intravenous formulations, without need for aseptic preparation. Finally, they share with transdermal systems the advantage that treatment can be rapidly stopped by removing the dose form.

Nevertheless, there are disadvantages. Absorption is passive, and so only small lipophilic molecules are well absorbed. Polar drugs are poorly absorbed, as are those which are highly ionised at the pH of the mouth (pH 6.2-7.4). Little intercellular absorption is possible across the cuboid squamous pavement epithe-lium of the oral cavity. The dose form must be kept in place while absorption is occurring since excessive salivary flow may wash it away. The taste of the drug must be bland, otherwise it will not be acceptable. The sublingual route is not suitable for the production of extended plasma concentration-time profiles, since absorption is completed quite quickly. The rate of dissolution of the formulation may be position dependent, due to variations in its proximity to the major salivary gland and the water content of the saliva produced.

Some drugs when presented sublingually are rapidly absorbed leading to high peak plasma concentrations since the epithelium in the area is very thin (approximately 100 μm). This may cause problems which can be overcome by delivering the drug to the thicker buccal mucosa which slows absorption. The tablet is placed between the cheek and the gum (e.g. in the upper buccal sulcus) and left in position for several hours. Initially the drug is absorbed rapidly, providing a quick onset of action, and subsequently there is slow continuous absorption for a few hours, during which time the effect of the drug should be maintained. This suggests that the buccal epithelium can act as a reservoir for administered drug after the delivery system has been removed, since back diffusion of a drug can occur if the mouth is washed out with a buffer of the correct pH (Davis and Johnston, 1979). Ideally the plasma concentration versus time profile should resemble a square wave, similar to that seen after skin application of a glyceryl trinitrate patch.

In order to be absorbed orally, the drug must first dissolve in the saliva. Extremely hydrophobic materials (those with partition coefficients greater than approximately 2000) will not dissolve well and are likely to be swallowed intact unless a specialized delivery system is used to present them to the mucosa. Saliva containing dissolved drug is constantly being swallowed, and this process competes with buccal absorption. As with many situations in which a drug is dissolved in a biological fluid prior to absorption, a compromise must be found between good dissolution (implying a large ionised fraction of drug) and a large unionised fraction of drug (implying poor solubility). Drugs with low partition coefficients are not well absorbed because they are too water soluble and cannot provide a suitable concentration of unionised species to partition into the plasma membrane. However, adequate concentrations in the saliva cannot be obtained if the partition coefficient is too high. A partition coefficient range of 40-2000 has been found to be optimal for drugs to be used sublingually. The importance of partition can be seen in the absorption of p-substituted phenylacetic acids, in order of increasing hydrophobicity, all of which have approximately the same pKa, the buccal absorption at pH 6 are: hydrogen - 1%, nitro - 1%, methoxy - 3%, methyl-7%, ethyl -10%, t-butyl - 25%, n-butyl - 34% n-pentyl - 49%, cyclohexyl - 44% and n-hexyl -61% (Beckett and Moffat, 1969).

Differences in Permeability Across the Oral Mucosa

Variations in surface layer thickness and composition will undoubtedly affect drug absorption. The permeability of the oral mucosa has been reviewed by Squier and Johnson (1975). The usual test of buccal absorption measures the average value of penetration of drug through all the different regions of the oral mucosa, even though it is likely that regional differences in absorption occur. It has been suggested that drug absorption through the sublingual mucosa is more effective than through the buccal mucosa, even though both these regions are non-keratinised. The sublingual epithelium is, however, thinner and immersed in saliva, both of which will aid drug absorption (Figure 2.6).

Squier and Rooney (1976) and Kaaber (1973) have demonstrated that keratinised

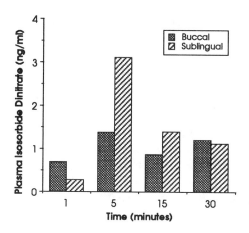

Figure 2.6. - Comparison of ISDN absorption when drug is presented by the buccal/sublingual route (after Pimlott and Addy, 1985)

and non-keratinised oral epithelia are equally impermeable to electrolytes which, like peroxidase, tend to pass through the intracellular space. Intercellular junctions do not appear to affect the permeability of these tissues unlike other epithelia. It was postulated by Squier and Johnson (1975) that the presence of the intercellular barrier did not correspond to the the distribution of the keratinised and non-keratinised layers, but more importantly to the presence of membrane-coating granules. These organelles are absent from junctional epithelia and at the gingival margin, the areas of highest permeability. Generally, molecules penetrate more readily than ions, small molecules more readily than large ones and volatile substances and gases to the greatest extent. However, dextrans with a molecular weight up to 70,000 will cross non-keratinised rabbit mucosa *in vitro* (Tolo and Jonsen, 1975).

The gingival sulcus is lined on its external surface by oral sulcular epithelium, which is continuous with the oral epithelium, but it is non-keratinised and has similar permeability to the oral epithelium (Figure 2.7). However, the "leakiest" area of the

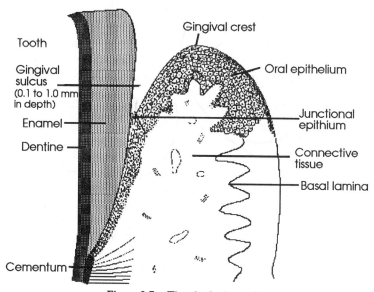

Figure 2.7. - The gingival margin

oral mucosa is the junctional epithelium in the gingival sulcus. This area has been studied extensively with respect to inflammatory periodontal disease. It is well documented that enzymes, toxins and antigens from plaque enter into the local tissue through this route and produce an immune inflammatory response in the tissue. Radioisotope and fluorescent compounds injected systemically can be detected at the surface. In healthy people, the sulcus is shallow or non-existent, and its base is formed by junctional epithelium, which extends from the base of the sulcus. The intercellular spaces in the junction epithelium are considerably larger than in either the oral sulcular epithelium or the oral epithelium and desmosome attachment is four times less common. The sulcus produces a fluid which is composed of an inflammatory exudate (reviewed by Cimasoni, 1974). Mild mechanical agitation of the surface of the sulcular epithelium increases the flow of gingival fluid, and many workers believe that no fluid flow occurs if the tissue is undisturbed, both in healthy and inflamed states.

Studies which have been carried out to examine the penetration of materials into the body via this route have rarely distinguished between junctional epithelium and oral sulcular epithelium and many animals have a different epithelial attachment to man. Substances which have been claimed at various times to penetrate the sulcular epithelium are albumin, endotoxins, thymidine, histamine and horse-radish peroxidase, which indicates a permeability of substances up to a molecular weight of 1 million (Squier and Johnson, 1975). Particulate material such as polystyrene microspheres between 1 - 3 μm in diameter have been reported to penetrate the epithelium (Fine *et al.*, 1969). It has been suggested (McDougall, 1971, 1972) that substances entering the gingiva do so through the intercellular spaces. Topically applied peroxidase was found in the intercellular spaces after 10 minutes. Application of hyaluronidase, which increases intercellular space, causes increased tracer uptake (Stallard and Awwa, 1969).

Gingival disease and aging are likely to influence drug absorption through the buccal cavity as the gum margin may recede or become inflamed allowing more access to the underlying connective tissues which limit only the passage of very large molecules, playing little part in the barrier function as a whole.

MEASUREMENT OF ORAL DRUG ABSORPTION.
The original buccal absorption test was introduced by Beckett and Triggs (1967). The subject is given the drug as an oral solution; after a measured period the mouth is emptied and rinsed, and the amount of unabsorbed drug remaining is assayed. This method has several disadvantages, primarily that an absorption-time profile must be built up from several separate experiments. The drug concentration also changes due to salivary secretion (Dearden and Tomlinson, 1971) and swallowing; this latter can be compensated by using a nonabsorbed internal marker (Schurmann and Turner, 1978). More recently Tucker (1988) has described a modification of the method which uses continuous oral sampling so that repeated experiments are not necessary. All these procedures suffer from the drawback that only absorption from the whole oral epithelia can be measured.

Kaaber (1973) used a gravimetric method for measuring the uptake or loss of water, sodium and potassium ions using a small filter paper discs applied to the mucosal surface, the ionic concentrations were determined by flame photometry. This method has the advantage that the absorption could be measured in specific regions of the oral mucosa. Veillard and coworkers (1987) described a chamber which could be applied to various regions of the mucosa and drug solution could be circulated through it. Plasma levels and effluent from the chamber could be analysed for drug content. This is a more elegant method of measuring drug absorption from the various regions of the mucosa.

DRUGS ADMINISTERED BY THE BUCCAL ROUTE
The buccal route has been explored for many drugs:
(1) Organic nitrates (nitroglycerin, isosorbide dinitrate) have been widely studied (e.g. Nyberg 1986, Ryden and Schaffrath 1987). GTN was rapidly absorbed (30 to 60 s) from 2.5 to 5 mg buccal doses and was more effective than a 10 mg transdermal patch. It was shown to be effective in prolonging the time to angina pectoris during exercise after a single dose, the effect lasting about five hours. Less convincing was its beneficial effect on heart failure in elderly patients in an open study over a minimum of fourteen days. Long-term therapy with buccal or transdermal glyceryl trinitrate may be associated with tolerance to the actions of the drug in association with sustained high plasma concentrations. A study by Ryden and Schaffrath (1987) reported that buccal nitroglycerin has a more pronounced prophylactic effect for the treatment of angina pectoris than sublingual nitroglycerin due to its longer duration of action, whereas both routes are comparable in the treatment of acute attacks.

2) Steroids such as deoxycorticosterone are absorbed through the oral mucosa, but a threefold increase in dosage over i.m. injections was required (Anderson *et al.*, 1940). Testosterone and methyltestosterone are more efficiently absorbed than by the peroral route (Miescher and Gasche, 1942; Escamilla and Bennett, 1951).

3) Opioids (morphine, pethidine) are well absorbed with systemic availability similar to that after intramuscular administration. Bell and coworkers (1985) demonstrated a substantial reduction in postoperative pain with buccally admini-stered morphine, comparable to that produced by the same dose of morphine given intramuscularly (Figure 2.8). Bioavailability and plasma concentrations of mor-phine has been reported to be higher after buccal than after intramuscular admini-stration (Bargett *et al.*, 1984). A study of fifty patients (Fisher *et al.*, 1986) undergoing various general surgical procedures demonstrated that buccal morphine was not as effective as intramuscular morphine in relieving preoperative anxiety and wakefulness. A later study by this group demonstrated that intramuscular administration of morphine produced an 8 fold increase in plasma levels compared to when the drug was administered buccally (Fisher *et al.*, 1987).

4) Calcium channel blockers (nifedipine, verapamil) both produce effects similar to oral doses when administered sublingually or buccally (Asthana *et al.*, 1984; Robinson *et al.*, 1980).

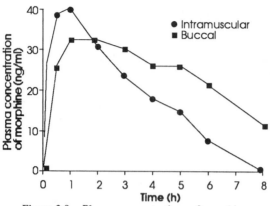

Figure 2.8. - Plasma concentrations of morphine following intramuscular and buccal routes of administration

5) Oxytocin was delivered by the buccal route (Miller, 1974), but this is now not often used since absorption was found to be variable, and it was of real benefit only when the cervix was already ripe. Its use has therefore been largely abandoned in favour of the intravenous route.

The buccal route has been tried with variable success for several other drugs, including ergotamine, isosorbide, phenazocine, propranolol, thyrotropin-releasing hormone, salbutamol, fenoterol and insulin. Recently, the buccal route has been explored for the delivery of peptides, and preliminary work in dogs demonstrated significant absorption of hydrophobic lauroyl derivative of a tripeptide (Veillard *et al.*, 1987).

DOSAGE FORMS FOR THE ORAL CAVITY
Chewable Formulations
Chewable formulations are used for the delivery of antacids where the flavouring agents give the sensation of relief and such a system may be preferred by the patient who has difficulty in swallowing tablets or capsules. The most important physiological variable is likely to be whether the subject sucks or chews the formulation. The rate of release of $^{99}Tc^m$ - DTPA from such formulations has been monitored *in vivo* in a group of volunteers who either sucked or chewed capsules containing various excipients (Figure 2.9). The results illustrated the marked effect on

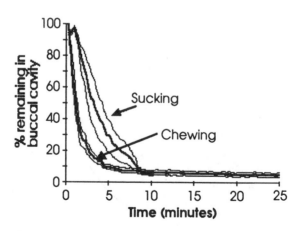

Figure 2.9. - Release of a radiolabelled marker from a chewable formulation (± s.d.)

dissolution of chewing the capsule. Systems which have been designed to be chewed will invariably be sucked by a proportion of patients and vice versa.

It has been discovered that smokers self-titrate the amount of nicotine which they are absorbing and hence a chewable nicotine formulation was devised to help people trying to withdraw from the habit. The theory was they chewed the gum until they has absorbed the correct amount of nicotine, then the formulation could be discarded. It has been of some value as a substitute to alleviate withdrawal symptoms during the transition period of giving up smoking (Mulry, 1988).

Christrup and coworkers (1988) have shown increased urinary recovery of vitamin C delivered in a chewing gum formulation, compared to the same dose given in a tablet. The abuse potential of narcotic drugs is reduced in this type of formulation since it is much harder to extract the active ingredient from the base for subsequent intravenous administration. The use of this type of formulation is being researched by the Royal Danish School of Pharmacy.

Fast-Dissolving Dosage Forms

Fast dissolving dose forms for analgesics are well established as convenient systems for patient dosing e.g. Solmin®. Recently a new type of dosage form (FDDF) based on a freeze-dried mixture of drug and fast-dissolving excipients has been introduced to deliver sedative drugs such as benzodiazepines. FDDFs are solid dose forms which do not have to be taken with water and are useful where swallowing is difficult or oesophageal clearance is impaired. Incorporation of technetium-99m labelled micronised "Amberlite" CG400 resin during manufacture enabled the deposition and clearance of these formulations to be followed by gamma scintigraphy (Wilson *et al.*, 1987). Two marker loadings were used, 2.5 mg and 10 mg, and the effect of incorporating the salivary stimulants talin/saccharin and citrate investigated.

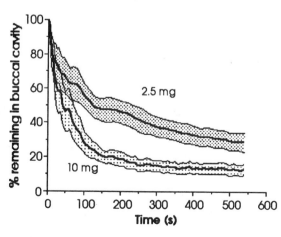

Figure 2.10. - Clearance of micronised resin from the tongue, trapping between the papallae (± s.d.)

It was noted that the buccal clearance of the formulation containing the 10 mg resin was significantly faster than that containing 2.5 mg resin (Figure 2.10); however, calculation of the total activity remaining after dissolution showed that the amount remaining on the tongue was approximately 1 mg in each case. This probably represents the amount of resin trapped within the papillae of the tongue. There was little spread of the formulation laterally in the buccal cavity.

Incorporation of salivary stimulants made little difference to the rate of dissolution of the formulation (Figure 2.11). This was not unexpected since salivary stimulants increase the output of the submandibular and sublingual salivary glands, which discharge watery secretions onto the floor of the mouth, wetting the side of the tongue and cheek surfaces. The posterior third of the tongue surface contains mucus glands, but the quantity of secretion is relatively small. Thus increased saliva flow may not result in more aqueous phase available for dissolution of the dosage form from the tongue surface. Delivery of drugs from a fast-dissolving formulation would not be expected to avoid first-pass metabolism since the unit disintegrated rapidly and the drug would be swallowed.

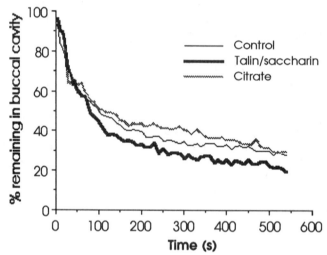

Figure 2.11. - Lack of an effect of salivary stimulants on dissolution of a fast dissolving dosage form

Bioadhesive Dosage Forms
Much interest has been shown in the extension of the transdermal principles to achieve drug flow through the buccal membranes by placing a covered patch at various sites in the mouth. This permits the local alteration of pH and inclusion of permeation enhancers which can markedly increase transport of drug. The use of the covered system removes luminal influences, such as saliva, mucus and enzymes, but keratinisation, the presence of intercellular lipids, the thickness and the blood supply then become rate limiting.

One of the newer formulations is a buccal or transmucosal tablet of glyceryl trinitrate which is placed between the teeth and the inside of the lips. The surface of the tablet quickly gels and serves both to anchor the tablet in position and to control the rate of diffusion of the drug. The tablet is based on a matrix of modified hydroxypropylmethylcellulose (Schor, 1980). Gamma scintigraphy was used to study the inter- and intra-subject variation (Figure 2.12), the effect of position in the buccal cavity and of chewing and drinking on the rate of release of $^{99}Tc^m$ DTPA from the tablet (Davis *et al.*, 1983). The tablets are friable and the gel layer breaks on removal, and the advantage of gamma scintigraphy is that the *in situ* dissolution can be measured without disturbing the tablet. When the tablet was placed in the upper buccal pouch it was noted that between subjects there were marked differences in the rates of release, whereas within an individual measured on four occasions, the variation was quite small. This did not appear to be

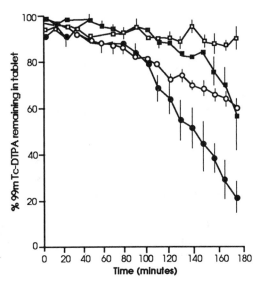

Figure 2.12. - Inter and intra-subject variation in rates of release of marker from a buccal dosage form

due to differences in saliva flow rate and the rate of dissolution may correlate with the extent to which the subject talked during the experiment. Articulation of the cheek surfaces during speech would increase the erosion of the tablet surface and hence the rate of release of the marker or drug into the buccal cavity.

The rate of release of marker did not increase when the subject drank hot coffee or chewed gum. In general, when the the tablet was placed behind the front incisors the rate of release of the technetium-99m marker was faster than when it was placed in the buccal cavity (Figure 2.13). Jenkins and Krebsbach (1985) have measured the path of saliva flow in the human mouth by monitoring the path of charcoal particles placed at various locations. When the particles were placed under the tongue, the whole mouth became covered within 1 to 3 minutes, whereas administration to the lower right or left buccal vestibule covered that side of the tongue only. Hence,

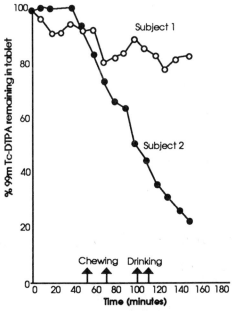

Figure 2.13. - Effect of chewing and drinking on rate of release from a buccal dosage form

it is possible that saliva flow was responsible for the different rates of dissolution observed for the tablet.

Descriptions of a "semi-topical" buccal/gingival delivery system have recently appeared in the literature (Nagai and Konishi, 1987). These workers describe the formulation of lidocaine in a oral mucoadhesive tablet for the relief of toothache or prostaglandin PGF2α into a gingival plaster for orthodontic tooth removal. Gingival absorption of lidocaine was poor due to the relatively low pH caused by the presence of carbopol-934 and more lipophilic derivatives such as dibucaine are suggested as drug candidates. Studies in monkeys showed good results with the prostaglandin and limited clinical tests showed accelerated orthodontic tooth removal in 70% of patients studied.

Dental Systems
A controlled release compact containing tetracycline has been developed for treatment of severe forms of the diseases such as gingivitis, acute necrotising gingivitis, periodontitis and periodontosis (Collins *et al.*, 1989). The compacts (5 mm in diameter) were bonded to an upper molar and designed to release drug over a period of 10 days. The tetracycline was found to reduce the quantity of plaque and gingival inflammation produced by the bacterial toxins around the gum margin. It is possible that similar systems can be developed to take advantage of the "leakiest" part of the buccal mucosa, the junctional epithelium.

CONCLUSIONS
The attractiveness of this route of dosing is the avoidance of first-pass metabolism of drugs. Drugs which can successfully be delivered by this route need to be highly active and are able to produce a pharmacological response in small amounts. Absorption appears to be somewhat erratic due to an unpredictable salivary flow washing drug into the stomach, which is then available for absorption via the small intestine, and possibly the degree of plaque formation in the mouth and hence variability in junctional epithelium exposed. Routine use of the buccal route of drug administration has little to commend it in preference to more conventional routes for either short-term or long-term therapy.

REFERENCES
Anderson E., Haymaker W. and Henderson E. (1940) Successful sublingual therapy in Addison's disease. *J. Am. Med. Assoc.* **115** 216-217.

Asthana O.P., Woodcock B.G., Wenchel M., Frömming K.H., Schwabe L. and Rietbrock N. (1984) Verapamil disposition and effects on PQ intervals after buccal, oral and intravenous administration. *Drug Res.* **34** 498-502.

Bardgett D., Howard C., Murray G.R., Calvey T.N. and Williams N.E. (1984) Plasma concentration and bioavailability of buccal preparation of morphine sulphate. *Br. J. Clin. Pharmacol.* **17** 198P-199P

Beckett A.H. and Moffatt A.C. (1969) The influence of substitution in phenyl acetic acids on their performance in the buccal absorption test. *J. Pharm. Pharmacol.* **21** 139S.

Beckett A.H. and Triggs E.R. (1967) Buccal absorption of basic drugs and its application as an *in vivo* model of passive drug transfer through lipid membranes. *J. Pharm.*

Pharmacol. **19** 31S-41S.

Bell M.D.D., Murray G.R., Mishra P., Calvey T.N., Weldon B.D. and Williams N.E. (1985) Buccal morphine - a new route for analgesia? *Lancet* i 71-73.

Christrup L.L., Rasmussen S.N. and Rassing M.R. (1988) Chewing gum as a drug delivery system. *Proc. 3rd International Conference on Drug Absorption*, Edinburgh.

Cimasoni G. (1974) Monographs in oral science, *The crevicular fluid.* 3 Karger, Basel.

Collins A.E.M., Deasy P.B., MacCarthy D.J. and Shanley D.B. (1989) Evaluation of a controlled-release compact containing tetracycline hydrochloride bonded to a tooth for the treatment of periodontal disease. *Int. J. Pharmaceut.* **51** 103-114.

Davis B.J. and Johnston A. (1979) Buccal absorption of verapamil - evidence for membrane storage. *Br. J. Clin. Pharmacol.* **7** 434P

Davis S.S., Kennerley J.W., Taylor M.J., Hardy J.G. and Wilson C.G. (1983) Scintigraphic studies on the *in vivo* dissolution of a buccal tablet. In *Modern Concepts in Nitrate Delivery Systems*. Ed. Goldberg A.A.J and Parsons D.G. Royal Society of Medicine. International Congress and Symposium Series No. 54 pp29-37.

Dearden J.C. and Tomlinson E. (1971) Correction for effect of dilution on diffusion through a membrane. *J. Pharm. Sci.* **60** 1278 - 1279.

Escamilla R.F. and Bennett L.L. (1951) Pituitary infantilism treated with purified growth hormone, thyroid and sublingual methyltestosterone. Case report. *J. Clin. Endocrinol.* **11** 221-228.

Fine D.H., Pechersky J.L. and McKibben D.H. (1969) The penetration of human gingival sulcular tissue by carbon particles. *Arch. Oral Biol.* **14** 1117-1119.

Fisher A.P., Vine P., Whitlock J. and Hanna M. (1986) Buccal morphine premedication. *Anaesthesia* **41** 1104-1111.

Fisher A.P., Fung C. and Hanna M. (1987) Serum morphine concentrations after buccal and intramuscular morphine administration. *Br. J. Clin. Pharmacol.* **24** 685-687.

Jenkins G.N. and Krebsbach P.M. (1985) Experimental study of the migration of charcoal particles in the human mouth. *Arch. Oral Biol.* **30** 697-699.

Kaaber S. (1973) Studies on the permeability of human oral mucosa. vi. The mucosal transport of water, sodium and potassium under varying osmotic pressure. *Acta Odont. Scand.* **31** 307-316.

McDougall W.A. (1971) Penetration pathways of a topically applied foreign protein into rat gingiva. *J. Periodontal Res.* **6** 89-99.

McDougall W.A. (1972) Ultrastructural localisation of antibody to an antigen applied topically to rabbit gingiva. *J. Periodontal Res.* **7** 304-314.

Miescher K. and Gasche P. (1942) Zur lingualen Applikation von männlichem sexualhormon; Beitrag zur Therapie mit "Perandren-Linguetten". *Schweiz. Med. Wochenschr.* **72** 279-281.

Miller G.W. (1974) Induction of labour by buccal administration of oxytocin. *J. Am. Osteopath. Assoc.* **72** 1110-1113.

Mulry J.T. (1988) Nicotine gum dependency: a positive addiction. *Drug Intell. Clin. Pharm.* **22** 313-314.

Nagai T. and Konishi R. (1987) Buccal/gingival drug delivery systems. *J. Cont.rolled Release* **6** 353-360.

Nyberg G. (1986) Onset time of action and duration up to 3 hours of nitroglycerin in buccal, sublingual and transdermal form. *Europ. Heart J.* **7** 673-678.

Pimlott S.J. and Addy.M. (1985) A study into the mucosal absorption of isosorbide dinitrate at different intraoral sites. *Oral Surg. Oral Med. Oral Path.* **59** 145-148.

Robinson B.F., Dobbs R.J., and Kelsey C.R. (1980) Effects of nifedipine on resistance of vessels, arteries and veins in man. *Br. J. Clin. Pharmacol.* **10** 433-438.

Ryden L. and Schaffrath R. (1987) Buccal versus sublingual nitroglycerin administration in the treatment of angina pectoris: a multi centre study. *Europ. Heart J.* **8** 994-1001

Schor J.M.(1980) Sustained release therapeutic compositions. U.S. Patent 4226849.

Schurmann W. and Turner P. (1978) A membrane model of the human oral mucosa as derived from buccal absorption performance and physicochemical properties of the beta-blocking drugs atenolol and propranolol. *J. Pharm. Pharmacol.* **30** 137-147.

Shannon I.L. and Prigmore J.R. (1958) Physiologic chloride levels in human whole saliva. *Proc. Soc. Exptl. Biol. Med.* **97** 825-828.

Sobrero A. (1847) Surplusiers composé détonants produit avec l'acide nitrique et le sucre, la dextrine, la lactine, la mannite et la glycérine. *Comptes, Rendus Hebdomadaires des Séances de l'Academie des Sciences* **24** 247-248.

Squier C.A. and Johnson N.W. (1975) Permeability of oral mucosa. *Br. Med. Bull.* **31** 169-175.

Squier C.A. and Rooney L. (1976) The permeability of keratinised and non-keratinised oral epithelium to lanthanum *in vivo. J. Ultrastruct. Res.* **54** 286-295.

Stallard R.E. and Awwa I.A. (1969) The effect of alterations in external environment on dento-gingival junction. *J. Dent. Res.* **48** 671-675.

Tolo K.J. and Jonsen B.J. (1975) *In vitro* penetration of tritiated dextrans through rabbit oral mucosa. *Arch. Oral Biol.* **20** 419-422.

Tucker I.G. (1988) A method the study the kinetics of oral mucosa drug absorption from solutions. *J. Pharm. Pharmacol.* **40** 679-683.

Veillard M.M., Longer M.A., Martens T.W. and Robinson J.R. (1987) Preliminary studies of oral mucosal delivery of peptide drugs. *J. Controlled Release* **6** 123-131.

Wilson C.G., Washington N., Peach J.M., Murray G.R. and Kennerley J. (1987) The behaviour of a fast dissolving dosage form (Expidet) followed by gamma scintigraphy. *Int. J. Pharmaceut.* **40** 119-123.

3

Oesophageal Transit

The oesophagus serves to move boluses of food, drink or drug formulations from the buccal cavity through the cardia into the stomach. Contact with the oesophageal tissue is normally very short, although certain pathological conditions can cause prolonged retention of a food bolus or dosage form. Posture also appears to be important. Taking a tablet whilst recumbent may have the advantage of increased compliance, but may decrease the rate of oesophageal transit with the risk of iatrogenic disease caused by the formulation, as will be demonstrated in this chapter.

The appreciation that oesophageal transit of formulations could be a major problem appears to stem from the introduction of wax-based matrix tablets of potassium chloride (Pemberton, 1970). Kikendall and co-workers (1983) reviewed the literature on "pill-induced" oesophageal injury over a period from 1960 to 1981 and reported on the data from 221 cases in 58 publications. Whilst most of the injuries were self-limiting and symptoms such as retrosternal pain and dysphagia were noted, there were instances of serious complications such as mediastinal perforation and haemorrhage leading to death. Additionally, retention of a formulation in the oesophagus can lead to reduced or delayed absorption of a drug (Channer and Roberts, 1985).

ANATOMY AND PHYSIOLOGY OF THE OESOPHAGUS
The oesophagus is a 25 cm long, 2 cm diameter muscular tube which joins the pharynx to the cardiac orifice of the stomach. The stratified squamous epithelium lining the buccal cavity is continued through the pharynx down into the oesophagus, but the lowest 2 cm or so of the oesophagus, which lies within the abdominal cavity, is normally lined with gastric mucosa and covered by peritoneum. The pH of the normal oesophageal lumen is usually between 5 and 6.

The oesophagus, stomach, small and large intestine have a common basic structure. The epithelium which lines the gastrointestinal tract is supported by the lamina propria. The muscularis mucosae is a thin layer of muscle which lies beneath the lamina propria and is responsible for local conformation of the overlying tissue. The external muscle consists of two bands: the inner circular and outer longitudinal layers.

The oesophagus has four coats, a fibrous external layer, a muscular layer, a submucous or areolar layer and an internal or mucous layer (Figure 3.1).

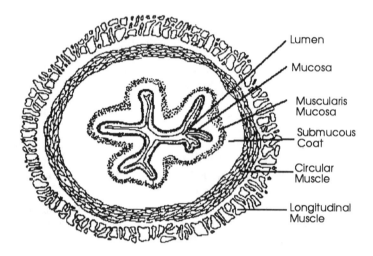

Figure 3.1. - Cross section through the oesophagus

i) The fibrous coat consists of elastic fibres embedded in a layer of areolar tissue.
ii) The muscular layer is composed of circular muscle surrounded by longitudinal muscle. Smooth muscle is found in the lower third of the oesophagus, striated muscle in the upper part and both types are found in the middle section.
iii) The areolar or submucous coat contains the larger blood vessels, nerves and mucous glands. It loosely connects the mucous and muscular coats.
iv) The mucosal layer consists of a layer of stratified squamous epithelium, one of connective tissue, and a layer of longitudinal muscle fibres, the *muscularis mucosae*. It forms longitudinal folds in its resting state which disappear when distended.

The main body of the oesophagus is lined with simple mucous glands, but towards the stomach they change from being simple glands to compound glands. The glands are small racemose glands of the mucous type and each opens into the lumen by a long duct which pierces the muscularis mucosae. The principal reason for secretion is to lubricate food and protect the lower part of the oesophagus from gastric acid.

The oesophagus possesses both sympathetic and parasympathetic innervation. Extrinsic innervation consists of a supply from the vagus nerves and sympathetic fibres derived from the cervical and thoracic ganglia. The intrinsic supply is derived from the Auerbach and Meissner plexuses. Neurites are found in the circular muscle of the oesophagus. They also run over the surface of interstitial cells which are not present in the longitudinal layer. These cells are called interstitial cells of Cajal and they possess a round or oval nucleus and a long, flat broad process which extends between the muscle. The precise function of these cells has not yet been discovered, but it is thought that they co-ordinate muscle contraction.

GASTRO-OESOPHAGEAL JUNCTION OR CARDIA.

The distal or lower oesophageal sphincter, also called the cardia, represents the transition between the oesophagus and the stomach. There is no precise definition of this area and it has been defined as 1) the junction of squamous and columnar epithelium, 2) the point at which the oesophagus enters the stomach, and 3) the junction between the oesophageal inner muscle layer and the inner layer of oblique muscle of the stomach (Figure 3.2). These features all occur in the human stomach within 1 cm of each other. The definition by manometry is a high pressure zone, 2 to 6 cm in length, with an intraluminal pressure of 15 to 40 mm Hg above intragastric pressure. The sphincter prevents gastro-oesophageal

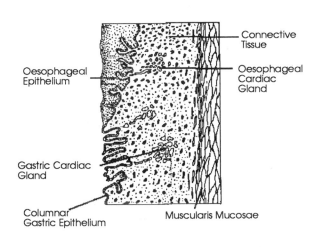

Figure 3.2. - Transverse section through the cardia

reflux, i.e. acidic gastric contents from reaching stratified epithelia of the oesophagus, where they can cause inflammation and irritation. The major problem with this theory is that in man no muscular sphincter has been conclusively identified.

MOTILITY OF THE OESOPHAGUS

The resting pressure in the oesophagus reflects the changes due to breathing which cause cycles of positive and negative intrathoracic pressure between -5 to -10 mm Hg (Torr) during inspiration, to 0 to +5 mm Hg during expiration. After a swallow, a single peristaltic wave of contraction passes the length of the oesophagus at the rate of 2 to 6 cm per second, gradually becoming faster at the lower end (Figure 3.3). The peak of the wave is usually above 40 mm Hg, but there is considerable intra-subject variation. If a second swallow is taken before the peristaltic wave from the

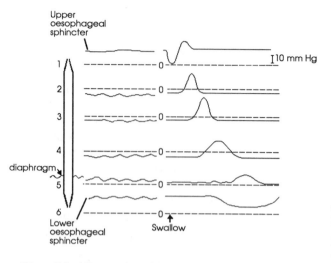

Figure 3.3. - Progression of a peristaltic wave through the oesophagus

first swallow has reached the base of the oesophagus, then the initial peristaltic wave is interrupted by the second peristaltic wave. When swallows are repeated in quick succession, then the contraction of the oesophagus is inhibited until the last swallow occurs; only the final peristaltic wave proceeds uninterrupted to the cardia carrying any food bolus or drug formulation with it (Ham *et al.*, 1985). In the upright position swallowing is assisted by gravity and this is prominent with liquids where the liquid travels faster than the peristaltic wave it has initiated. Secondary peristaltic waves arise from distension of the oesophagus and serve to move sticky lumps of food or refluxed materials into the stomach. Initiation of secondary peristalsis is involuntary and is not normally sensed. Variation in the size of the bolus being swallowed leads to a variation in the amplitude of oesophageal contraction.

OESOPHAGEAL TRANSIT

Oesophageal transit is usually assessed clinically by x-ray study of a swallowed bolus of barium sulphate suspension. A major problem with this is that barium sulphate is extremely dense and if the subject is in the upright position, its transit will be considerably affected by gravity. The transit of heavy capsules is considerably faster than transit of light capsules (Channer and Virjee, 1985a). Barium has been used to assess oesophageal transit of cylinders of gelatin (Mickey, 1929), marshmallows (McNally and Del Gaudio, 1967; Kelly, 1961), cotton pledgets, tablets (Wolf, 1961; Evans and Roberts, 1976) and capsules (Schatzki and Gary, 1953). X-ray contrast techniques are difficult to quantify and are associated with a significant radiation burden on the subjects. Recently, gamma scintigraphy has been used to assess oesophageal transit since it is capable of following any suitably labelled test material, food or dosage forms. The transit can be expressed as position of radioactivity against time (Figure 3.4).

The oesophageal transit of dose forms is extremely rapid, usually of the order of 10 to 14 seconds. Typical times for transit of pharmaceutical dosage forms are shown in Table 3.1.

This data suggests that the size and shape of formulations only has a small effect when compared to the influence of the posture of the subject. Large oval tablets have a shorter oesophageal transit than large round tablets as might be expected, but there is little clear agreement whether capsules are more prone to adhesion than tablets. In all studies, the number of formulations lodging in the oesophagus is increased when the subject is supine, with an approximately 20% incidence of adhesion.

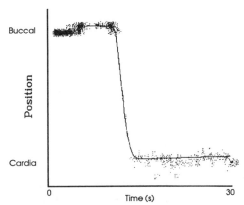

Figure 3.4. - Plot of position of activity versus time for a swallow of technetium-99m -DTPA labelled water.

Bolus Composition

Fisher and coworkers (1982) have studied the effect of bolus composition on oesophageal transit. They concluded that liquids cleared rapidly, with one swallow regardless of whether the subjects were supine or seated, but capsules or liver cubes when ingested without water, frequently remained in the oesophagus up to 2 hours after administration, without the subject being aware of their presence. Kjellén and

Table 3.1. - Mean transit times for pharmaceutical formulations through the oesophagus

Formulation Weight & Dimensions	Transit time (Median) (s)	Posture	Reference
Tablet 100mg Round 6mm Diameter,	13	Supine	(a)
Tablet Oval (14mm x 9mm) Film-coated	3	Erect	(b)
Tablet Oval (14mm x 9mm) Film-coated	>300	Supine	(b)
Tablet Oval (14mm x 9mm)	>300	Supine	(b)
Tablets (Various sizes & shapes)	8	Supine	(c)
Tablets (Various)	4	Erect	(d)
Capsule Hard gelatin, Size 2	10	Supine	(a)
Capsule Hard gelatin, Size 2 (0.59g)	10	Supine	(b)
Capsule Hard gelatin, Size 2 (1.2g)	80	Supine	(b)
Capsule Hard gelatin, Size 2 (0.59g)	9	Erect	(b)
Capsule Hard gelatin, Size 2 (1.2g)	3	Erect	(b)
Capsule Hard gelatin, Size 0 (1.2g)	3	Erect	(b)
Capsule Hard gelatin, Size 0 (1.2g)	45	Supine	(b)
Capsule Hard gelatin, Size 0 (0.67g)	9	Erect	(b)
Capsule Hard gelatin, Size 0 (1.2g)	9	Supine	(b)
Liquid, 20ml	10	Supine	(a)

(a) Wilson *et al.*, 1988, (b) Channer and Virjee 1985b, (c) Hey *et al.*, 1982,
(d) Channer and Virjee, 1986.

co-workers (1981a) studied a solid gelatin bolus with subjects seated; these workers measured a transit time of 6.6 ± 2.1 seconds (mean ± s.d.) with no mention of oesophageal sticking.

Effect of diseased states on transit

Oesophageal transit may be influenced by diseased states such as achalasia, in which transit is impaired by an oesophageal stricture or inability of the lower oesophageal sphincter to relax. Oesophageal retention of food results. Additionally, abnormalities in oesophageal function can occur as a result of a variety of diseased states such as diabetes mellitus, chronic alcoholism and scleroderma. Reflux of gastric contents can cause injury to the oesophageal mucosa and the oesophagitis produced can lead to stricture (Evans and Roberts, 1976, 1981). Oesophageal dysfunction has been shown to be more common in asthmatics than normal subjects (Kjellén et al., 1981b), so drugs such as theophylline may show an increased incidence of adhesion (D'Arcy, 1984).

ADHESION OF DOSAGE FORMS TO THE OESOPHAGUS

It is well recognised that tablets or capsules taken by patients in the supine position may lodge in the oesophagus causing damage and irritation (Channer and Virjee, 1982; Heller et al., 1982; Al-Dujaili et al., 1983; Fell, 1983) and it is now generally accepted that oesophageal transit is markedly affected by the posture of the subject and the amount of water used to swallow the dosage form. If tablets are taken without water the risk is greatly increased and the unit may remain lodged in the lower oesophagus until it disintegrates (Hey et al., 1982).

In a study of 50 subjects, Channer and Virjee (1982) compared the effect of 15 and 60 ml volumes taken with a hard gelatin capsule. Whilst standing, complete oesophageal transit was observed by 5 s when capsules were taken with 60 ml of water. In approximately 10% of patients taking a tablet with the smaller volume, the capsules stuck. If recumbent, the adhesion was more pronounced with 40% sticking in the 15 ml and 30% sticking in the 60 ml volume groups. Bailey and coworkers (1987) carried out a scintigraphic study on normal subjects, comparing a small and large volume of water, and measured oesophageal peristalsis by manometry. They reported that the subjects whose capsules lodged in the oesophagus with the large volume of water had lower mean amplitudes of contractions. The problem of adhesion of dosage forms to the mucosa can be aggravated in patients who have cardiac pathologies in which the left side of the heart is enlarged or who are elderly and have oesophageal dysfunction. Applegate and coworkers (1980) reiterate the early suggestion of Fisher and coworkers that capsules should taken with a "chaser" of at least 15 ml of water.

Mechanism of Adhesion

The interior surface of the oesophagus is moist rather than wet and a dosage form in contact with the mucosa will cause partial dehydration at the site of contact as the unit hydrates, resulting in formation of a gel between the formulation and the mucosa (Figure 3.5). The unit then disintegrates from its non-contact side. Disintegration of the lodged formulation is slow, firstly because the amount of dissolution fluid available is low, being dependent on the volume of swallowed saliva, and secondly due to the reduced surface area available for dissolution.

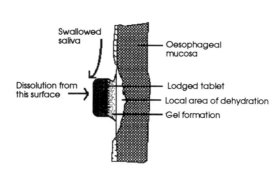

Figure 3.5. - Mechanism of adhesion of a tablet to the oesophageal mucosa.

Factors Predisposing Formulations to Adhere

In general, there are several factors which predispose a formulation to adhere:
a) shape of dosage form
b) size of dosage form
c) position of subject
d) volume of water with which the dosage form is administered
e) surface characteristics of the dosage form.

Large oval and large circular tablets have the greatest tendency to stick when subjects are in the supine position or when little water is administered (Wamberg *et al.*, 1983). Marvola and coworkers (1982) and Swisher and coworkers (1984) studied adhesion of dosage forms to isolated preparations of oesophagus and concluded that hard gelatin capsules had the greatest tendency to adhere, followed by film coated tablets, uncoated tablets, with sugar coated tablets demonstrating the least adhesion.

The hydration of a sticky material against the mucosal epithelium greatly increases the chances for adhesion and has been recognised as a hazard of formulations containing gelatin or cellulose derivatives (Swisher *et al.*, 1984). Hard gelatin capsules absorb water and become adherent to the mucosa if their passage is delayed for more than 2 minutes (Channer and Virjee, 1982). Fell (1983) has challenged the belief that gelatin capsules are more likely to stick than tablets, and concluded that both dosage forms should be regarded as having equal potential to adhere.

Tablets are often coated to render them more acceptable to the patient or to protect the drug from gastric acid etc., but the coatings themselves may affect the tendency for formulations to adhere. Channer and Virjee (1985b) showed that, although coated tablets had significantly shorter oesophageal transit times than plain tablets, the coated tablets were slower to disintegrate if they became lodged in the oesophagus. Coatings made from cellulose acetate phthalate, shellac, methacrylate copolymer and a copolymer composed of vinyl acetate and crotonic acid all have a low tendency to adhere. The tendency of hydroxypropylmethylcellulose to adhere can be adjusted by incorporation of sucrose which reduces surface stickiness; conversely addition of lactose or titanium oxide and talc increases the tendency to adhere (Marvola *et al.*, 1983). In contrast, polyethylene glycol 6000 coating demonstrated the greatest tendency to adhere.

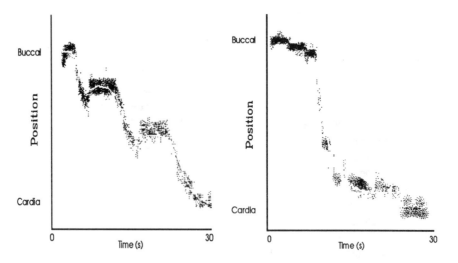

Figure 3.5. - Clearance of a fast-dissolving   Figure 3.6. - Clearance of a capsule
dosage form from the oesophagus   from the oesophagus

Frequency of Sticking

In a recent study carried out at Nottingham capsules and tablets were observed to lodge in the oesophagus in two out of ten (20%) of the subjects (Wilson *et al.*, 1988). This compares with 37 capsules lodging in 175 subjects (21%) in the Channer and Virjee (1986) study and 160 out of 726 (22%) swallows in the study by Hey and coworkers (1982). The Expidet® formulation (American Home Products) is a rapidly disintegrating solid dosage form which can be taken without water. The general pattern of buccal clearance of the fast dissolving dosage form (Figure 3.6) was either to dissolve rapidly in the mouth and hence was cleared with several swallows, or to pass through the oesophagus intact and this is compared to the behaviour of a capsule (Figure 3.7) (Wilson *et al.*, 1988). Prolonged oesophageal retention of this type of formulation if swallowed as an intact unit is unlikely since the unit requires only a small volume of liquid to disperse the incorporated solids. Data suggest that this solid dosage form appears to have overcome the usual problems of oesophageal retention of the conventional dosage form taken without water.

Oesophageal Damage

Oesophageal retention of a formulation containing an irritant drug can lead to damage to the mucosa, ulceration and even stricture or perforation. This is produced by a prolonged contact of the drug at high concentrations with the mucosa. Oesophageal ulceration has been reported for many drugs including emepronium bromide (Fellows *et al.*, 1982), some antibiotics (Collins *et al.*, 1979), theophylline (Enzenauer *et al.*, 1984) and non-steroidal anti-inflammatory drugs (Heller *et al.*, 1982). Doxycycline hyclate has frequently been reported to induce lesions in the oesophagus (e.g. Bokey and Hugh, 1975; Schneider, 1977), but doxycycline monohydrate appeared to produce less toxicity in cats, unless gastro-oesophageal reflux of acid occurred (Carlborg and Farmer, 1983). This caused the monohydrate to be converted to the highly ulcerogenic hydrochloride salt (Borgardus and Blackwood, 1979). In humans, this problem would be compounded since delayed transit is associated with hiatus hernia and gastro-oesophageal reflux. Retention of the dosage form in the oesophagus has been demonstrated to delay drug absorption, as drugs cannot easily pass through the stratified squamous epithelium of the oesophageal mucosa (Channer and Roberts, 1984, 1985).

CONCLUSIONS

Oesophageal adhesion of dosage forms is surprisingly common and can cause problems of local ulceration or delayed drug absorption. It is important to emphasise the correct method of swallowing tablets to patients.

REFERENCES

Al-Dujaili H., Salole E.G. and Florence A.T. (1983) Drug formulation and oesophageal injury. *Adv. Drug React. Ac. Pois. Rev.* **2** 235-256.

Applegate G.R., Malmud L.S., Rock E., Reilley J.R. and Fisher R.S. (1980) "It's a hard pill to swallow" or "Don't take it lying down". *Gastroenterology* **78** 1132.

Bailey R.T., Bonavina L., McChesney L., Spires K.J. and DeMeester T.R. (1987) Factors influencing the transit of a gelatin capsule in the oesophagus. *Drug Intell. Clin. Pharm.* **21** 282-285.

Bokey L. and Hugh T.B. (1975) Esophageal ulcerations associated with doxycycline therapy. *Med. J. Aust.* **1** 236-237.

Borgardus J.B. and Blackwood R.K. (1979) Dissolution rates of doxycycline free base and hydrochloride salts. *J. Pharm. Sci.* **68** 1183-1184.

Carlborg B. and Farmer J.C. (1983) Esophageal corrosion tests with doxycycline monohydrate tablets. *Curr. Therap. Res.* **34** 110-116.

Channer K.S. and Roberts C.J.C. (1984) Antipyrine absorption after delayed oesophageal capsule transit. *Br. J. Clin. Pharmacol.* **18** 250-253.

Channer K.S. and Roberts C.J.C. (1985) Effect of delayed esophageal transit on acetaminophen absorption. *Clin. Pharmacol. Ther.* **37** 72-76.

Channer K.S. and Virjee J.P. (1982) Effect of posture and drink volume on the swallowing of capsules. *Br. Med. J.* **285** 1702.

Channer K.S. and Virjee J.P. (1985a) The effect of formulation on oesophageal transit. *J. Pharm. Pharmacol.* **37** 126-129.

Channer K.S. and Virjee J.P. (1985b) Effect of surface coating of tablets on oesophageal transit. *Br. J. Pharm. Pract.* **7** 9-10.

Channer K.S. and Virjee J.P. (1986) The effect of size and shape of tablets on their oesophageal transit. *J. Clin. Pharmacol.* **26** 141-146.

Collins F.J., Matthews H.R., Baker S.E. and Strakova J.M. (1979) Drug induced oesophageal injury. *Br. Med. J.* **1** 1673-1676.

D'Arcy P.F. (1984) Oesophageal problems with tablets and capsules. *Pharmacy International.* **5** 109.

Enzenauer R.W., Bass J.W. and McDonnell J.T. (1984) Esophageal ulceration associated with oral theophylline. *N. Engl. J. Med.* **310** 261.

Evans K.T. and Roberts G.M. (1976) Where do all the tablets go? *Lancet* **ii** 1237-1239.

Evans K.T. and Roberts G.M. (1981) The ability of patients to swallow capsules. *J. Clin. Hosp. Pharm.* **6** 207-208.

Fell J.T. (1983) Oesophageal transit of tablets and capsules. *Am. J. Hosp. Pharm.* **40** 946-948.

Fellows I.W., Ogilvie A.L. and Atkinson M. (1982) Oesophageal stricture associated with emepronium bromide therapy. *Postgrad. Med. J.* **75** 43-44.

Fisher R.S., Malmud L.S., Applegate G., Rock E. and Lorber S.H. (1982) Effect of bolus composition on esophageal transit: concise communication. *J. Nucl. Med.* **23** 878-882.

Ham H.R., Georges B., Froideville J.L. and Piepsz A. (1985) Oesophageal transit of liquid: effects of single or multiple swallows. *Nucl. Med. Comm.* **6** 263-267.

Heller S.R., Fellows I.W., Ogilvie A.L. and Atkinson M. (1982) Non-steroidal anti-inflammatory drugs and benign oesophageal stricture. *Br. Med. J.* **285** 167-168.

Hey H., Jørgensen F., Sørensen K., Hasselbalch H. and Wamberg T. (1982) Oesophageal transit of six commonly used tablets and capsules. *Br. Med. J.* **285** 1717-1719.

Kelly J.E. (1961) The marshmallow as an aid to radiologic examination of the esophagus. *New Eng. J. Med.* **265** 1306-1307.

Kikendall J.W., Friedman A.C., Oyewole M. .A., Fleischer D and Johnson L.F. (1983) Pill-induced esophageal injury: case reports and a review of the medical literature. *Dig. Dis. Sci.* **28** 174-182.

Kjellén G., Svedberg J.B. and Tibbling L. (1981a) Computerised scintigraphy of oesophageal bolus transit in asthmatics. *Int. J. Nucl. Med. Biol.* **8** 153-158.

Kjellén G., Brundin A., Tibbling L. and Wranne B. (1981b) Oesophageal function in asthmatics. *Eur. J. Resp. Dis.* **62** 87-94.

Marvola M., Vahervuo K., Sothmann A., Marttila E. and Rajaniemi M. (1982) Development of a method for study of the tendency of drug products to adhere to the esophagus. *J. Pharm. Sci.* **71** 975-977.

Marvola M., Rajaniemi M., Marttila E., Vahervuo K. and Sothmann A. (1983) Effect of dosage form and formulation factors on the adherence of drugs to the oesophagus. *J. Pharm. Sci.* **72** 1034-1037.

McNally E.E. and Del Gaudio W. (1967) The radiopaque esophageal marshmallow bolus. *Am. J. Roentgenol. Rad. Therapy and Nuclear Med.* **101** 485-489.

Mickey P.M. (1929) Method for measuring lumen of the oesophagus. *Radiology* **13** 469-471.

Pemberton J. (1970) Oesophageal obstruction and ulceration caused by oral potassium therapy. *Br. Heart J.* **32** 267-268.

Schatzki R. and Gary J.E. (1953) Dysphagia due to diaphragm-like localised narrowing in the lower esophagus (lower esophageal ring). *Am. J. Roentgenol. Rad. Therapy and Nuclear Med.* **70** 911-922.

Schnieder R. (1977) Doxycycline esophageal ulcers. *Dig. Dis. Sci.* **22** 805-807.

Swisher D.A., Sendelbeck S.L. and Fara J.W. (1984) Adherence of various oral dosage forms to the oesophagus. *Int. J. Pharmaceut.* **22** 219-228.

Wamberg T., Jørgensen F., Hasselbalch H. and Hey H. (1983) The prejudgment of the oesophageal transfer of tablets and capsules. *Arch. Pharm. Chem. Sci. Ed.* **11** 24-31.

Wolf B.S. (1961) Use of half-inch barium tablet to detect minimal esophageal strictures. *J. Mt. Sinai Hosp.* **28** 80-82.

Wilson C.G., Washington N., Norman S., Greaves J.L., Peach J.M. and Pugh K. (1988) A gamma scintigraphic study to compare oesophageal clearance of "Expidet" formulations, tablets and capsules in supine volunteers. *Int. J. Pharm.* **46** 241-246.

4

The stomach: its role in oral drug delivery

The major function of the stomach is to temporarily store food and release it slowly into the duodenum. It processes the food to a semi-solid chyme which enables better contact with the mucous membrane of the intestine, thereby facilitating absorption of nutrients. The stomach reduces the risk of noxious agents reaching the absorption sites in the small intestine, firstly by a bacteriostatic action of the gastric juice and secondly by stimulation of the vomiting reflex. In addition to its reservoir function, the stomach is an important site of enzyme production. The stomach is located below the diaphragm, but its exact position varies with the volume of food ingested, posture, skeletal build, tone of abdominal muscles and state of adjacent viscera.

Contrary to popular belief, very little drug absorption occurs from the stomach; more significantly, it provides a barrier to the delivery and hence absorption of drugs by the small intestine. The motility patterns which are responsible for gastric emptying depend upon the nature and frequency of food intake and therefore are extremely variable within and between individuals. Under normal conditions in which food intake is not controlled, gastric emptying of orally administered formulations is unpredictable, which can lead to erratic bioavailability.

ANATOMY AND PHYSIOLOGY OF THE STOMACH

The stomach can be divided into four anatomical regions: fundus, body, antrum and pylorus, which have different physiological functions (Figure 4.1). The proximal stomach or fundus acts as a reservoir and adjusts to the increased volume during eating by relaxation of the fundal muscle fibres which allows distension of the greater curvature and fundus. This action, termed receptive relaxation, results in little change in intragastric pressure during filling.

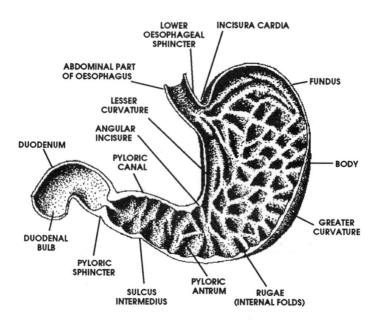

Figure 4.1. - Anatomy of the stomach

Liquid and solid emptying are controlled by the proximal and distal portions of the stomach respectively. The proximal stomach produces slow, sustained contractions which are responsible for the basal pressure in the stomach and it is thought that this pressure controls the gastric emptying of liquids. The second function of the fundus is to exert a steady pressure on the gastric contents, gradually pressing them towards the distal stomach. The distal portion or antrum of the stomach has a thicker, more muscular wall and it is concerned with the regulation of emptying of solids. The antrum acts as a homogeniser and grinder of food, breaking down the large particles and propelling the contents toward the pylorus for ejection into the duodenum as a milky, semi-solid chyme. The breaking up of food is more a mechanical process than an enzymatic one, although pepsin and acid begin to digest the protein component of the meal. This releases peptides causing reflex secretion of acid.

Gastric Mucosa

The entire mucosal surface of the stomach is lined with simple columnar epithelial cells and is chiefly concerned with the secretory process. The gastric mucosa is folded into rugae which possess numerous pits, at the base of which are simple branched tubular gastric glands. On average, a gastric pit contains four glands which are arranged perpendicularly to the surface (Figure 4.2). The body of the stomach is lined with mucous, parietal, peptic and G cells. The parietal (oxyntic) cells secrete acid and intrinsic factor, while the peptic (chief) cells secrete pepsinogen, the precursor for pepsin. The peptic cells are mainly located at the base of the gland, the parietal cells at the neck and isthmus and the mucous cells at the

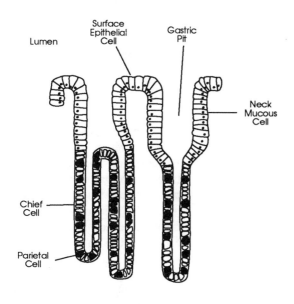

Figure 4.2. - Gastric pit containing chief and parietal cells

neck. G cells secrete gastrin and are mainly located in the surface epithelium in the mid-zone of the gastric glands.

The gastric mucosal cells are replaced by the mother or stem cells in the neck region of the gland. These are undifferentiated cells which migrate either towards the surface to form mucous cells, or into the gastric glands to form new peptic and parietal cells. The cells reach the surface in 2 to 3 days but movement into the pits is slower. The oldest cells are secreted into the gastric lumen and they are lost at the rate of 0.5×10^6 cells per minute.

Mucus and bicarbonate are secreted by the surface mucosal cells which line the mucosa, but are not found in the gastric glands. The pyloric area of the stomach possesses only mucus secreting cells. The bicarbonate and mucus protect the stomach from digestion by pepsin and the corrosive effects of hydrochloric acid. Mucus also has lubricating properties allowing chyme to move freely through the digestive system.

Gastric Secretion
Acid Secretion - Parietal cells are located in the mucosal glands and their distribution in the stomach is not uniform. A high concentration is present in the body of the stomach, relatively few in the fundus and none in the antrum. Parietal cells can secrete hydrogen ions at a concentration of 150 mmolar; in comparison, the H^+ concentration in blood is 40 nmolar. The pure parietal cell secretion is diluted to between 20 and 60 mmolar by non-parietal cell secretion. Normal adults produce a basal secretion up to 60 ml with approximately 4 mmol of H^+ per hour, which rises to more than 200 ml and 15 to 50 mmol H^+ when maximally stimulated.

Hydrogen ions are produced by metabolic activity in the parietal cells and this is summarised in Figure 4.3. The key reaction between water and carbon dioxide is catalysed by carbonic anhydrase. The bicarbonate ion produced diffuses back into the blood stream and after a meal is secreted in sufficient quantities to cause a rise in plasma pH and a marked alkalinity of urine, the "alkaline tide". The hydrogen

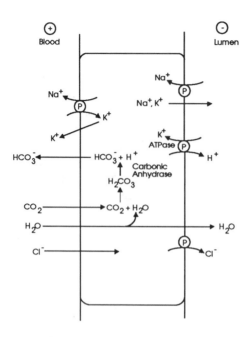

Figure 4.3. - Mechanism of acid secretion

ion is actively pumped into the stomach lumen in exchange for potassium ions. Potassium also diffuses passively out of the cell; pure parietal cell secretion is therefore a mixture of hydrochloric acid and potassium chloride.

Histamine is a potent stimulator of acid secretion and acts via the H_2 receptors which are concentrated on the gastric mucosa. Its precise role in the control of acid production has not yet been defined, but H_2 receptor antagonists, e.g. cimetidine, inhibit basal acid secretion and secretory responses to feeding, gastrin, histamine and vagal stimulation. An interesting finding has been that gastrin only weakly stimulates isolated parietal cells or gastric glands and this effect is insensitive to H_2 receptor blockade (Berglindh et al., 1976). It has been proposed that the powerful in vivo action of this hormone may be due to its release of histamine from gastric mucosa. Histamine containing cells must, therefore, have receptors to hormones such as gastrin, and vagal stimulation is believed to deliver transmitter directly to muscarinic receptors on the histamine containing cells (Angus, 1982).

Gastrin - The hormone gastrin is the most potent stimulator of gastric acid production. Its release is stimulated by peptides, amino acids and distension of the stomach. The pressure of food in the stomach stimulates mechano- and chemo-receptors in the mucosa. These receptors are especially sensitive to amino acids and related products of digestion and directly stimulate gastrin release from G-cells via local reflexes.

All the different forms of gastrin (big, little and mini) have the terminal tetrapeptide in common. The differences appear to be related to the distribution of the hormone in the tissues and plasma, biological activity, half-life, and circadian rhythm, especially in relation to the prandial or interprandial period.

Pepsins - Pepsins are secreted as their inactive precursors, pepsinogens. Acid autocatalytically cleaves inactive pepsinogens to active pepsins (molecular weight 34,000 Daltons) and also provides the optimum pH for pepsin activity. Pepsin can self-catalyse the formation of additional pepsin from pepsinogen. Pepsin activity is almost completely abolished above pH 5 as these enzymes are denatured at higher pH.

Human pepsins are endopeptidases, and hydrolyse several peptide bonds within the interior of ingested protein molecules to form polypeptides but little free amino acid. The most susceptible bonds involve the aromatic amino-acids, tyrosine or phenylalanine. The polypeptides produced have N-terminal amino acids with lipophilic side chains, which facilitate absorption. The pepsinogens and their corresponding pepsins have been classified by immunochemical techniques as PGI (pepsinogens 1-5) and PGII (pepsinogens 6-7). A high degree of correlation has been found between serum concentrations of PGI and maximal gastric acid secretion.

Other Enzymes - The stomach secretes small quantities of other enzymes such as gastric lipase, gastric amylase and gelatinase. Gastric lipase is a highly specific tributyrase, acting solely on butterfat which is tributyrin. Gastric amylase plays a minor role in the digestion of starches and the enzyme gelatinase helps liquify some of the proteoglycans in meats.

Intrinsic Factor of Castle - Parietal cells also secrete a glycoprotein of molecular weight 1350 Daltons known as intrinsic factor of Castle. Intrinsic factor, which is required for the absorption of vitamin B12 from the ileum, is continuously secreted in the absence of any gastric secretory stimuli in man and basal secretion greatly exceeds the minimum amount required for normal vitamin B12 absorption.

Mucus - Mucus is secreted by mucous cells which are concentrated in the neck of the gastric gland. The major components of mucus are galactose (33%), N-acetylglucosamine (31%) and fructose (21%), but the proportions of these may change in disease states such as ulceration. The mean thickness of the mucus in the human stomach is 140 μm. Mucus protects the gastric mucosa from autodigestion by the pepsin and acid combination present in the stomach (Figure 4.4). It contains bicarbonate ions which serve to raise the pH local to the epithelium

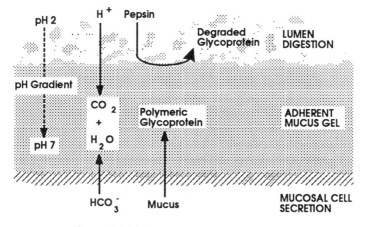

Figure 4.4. - Mucus degradation in the stomach

without raising the bulk pH and this produces additional protection by inactivating pepsin.

Mucus is continuously digested from the surface and replaced from beneath. The mucus turnover time, i.e. from production to digestion, is estimated to be between 4 to 5 hours. It is possible that the turnover time may be slower since mucous cells secrete copious amounts of mucus even after slight stimulation and so the measurement process may stimulate mucus production. Prostaglandins and carbachol approximately double the mean thickness of mucus and increase the amount of bicarbonate present.

Effect of food on gastric secretion
A normal adult has average daily intake of 3 to 4 kg of food and drink but an additional 5 litres of fluids such as saliva, gastric and pancreatic juice and other body fluids are secreted into the gut in response to this stimulation.

The greatest secretory activity occurs within the first hour of eating, and the volume produced may be up to twice that of the meal. The cephalic phase, initiated by the thought of food, followed by the sight, small and taste of the food, contributes approximately one third to one half of the acid secreted in response to food. This is mediated by the vagus nerve which directly stimulates parietal cells and increases the release of the hormone gastrin, which also has a potent acid secretory effect The cephalic phase is followed by the gastric phase of secretion, which is stimulated directly by the food and the distension produced by the stomach contents. Food, especially peptides and amino acids, stimulate gastrin release, but acidification of the antral mucosa to below pH 3 inhibits the gastrin release produced in response to digested protein. A distinct pH gradient exists in the stomach after a meal; the contents of the body of the stomach are neutralised, but this does not extend to the antrum, which remains relatively acid (Bumm and Blum, 1987; McLauglan *et al.*, 1989). Maintaining the antrum at a low pH serves as an inhibitory feedback mechanism for controlling the meal-stimulated release of gastrin. The presence of food in the duodenum causes the duodenal mucosa to release small amounts of gastrin which stimulates the stomach to secrete small quantities of acid.

The major physiological stimulus for acid secretion is the ingestion of food, especially if the meal has a high protein content. Interestingly, it is the protein component of the meal which possesses the greatest buffering capacity. The buffering action of food usually produces an initial increase in pH. In our studies, we have found the resting pH of healthy people to be around 1.8. A meal can increase the pH to between 3 and 5, but foods such as milk can raise gastric pH to over 6. The median daytime pH for eight subjects over a 24 hour period was 2.7 (range 1.8 to 4.5) in the body of the stomach and 1.9 (range 1.6 to 2.6) in the antrum (Figure 4.5) (McLauglan *et al.*, 1989). The preprandial pH for the two regions were similar, but the difference in the median pH observed was due to the different pH curves produced after meals. On commencing to eat, the pH in the body rose after

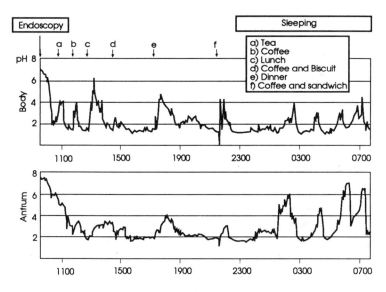

Figure 4.5. - pH in the body and antrum of the stomach in a healthy volunteer over a 24 hour period (after McLauglan *et al.*, 1989)

approximately 30 seconds (range 8-60 seconds) which was earlier than the antral pH which began to rise after 6 minutes (range 2-30 minutes). The time for the pH to return to preprandial levels was approximately 2 hours for both regions of the stomach. The difference in pH observed demonstrates that different patterns of motility exist between the body and antrum.

GASTRIC MOTILITY

The stomach is composed of two main layers of smooth muscle. The outer longitudinal muscle is in continuity with the duodenal muscle layer, while the inner circular layer extends only up to the pylorus (Figure 4.6). The stomach has a third oblique layer which appears to be in continuity with the muscle of the lower oesophageal sphincter. This arrangement of muscles allows the stomach to produce co-ordinated movements of the gastric contents.

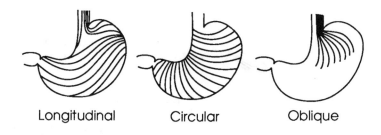

Figure 4.6. - Muscle layers of the stomach

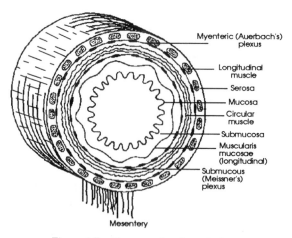

Myenteric (Auerbach's)
plexus

Longitudinal
muscle

Serosa

Mucosa

Circular
muscle

Submucosa

Muscularis
mucosae
(longitudinal)

Submucous
(Meissner's)
plexus

Mesentery

Figure 4.7. - Cross section through the gut

Two major nerves connect the stomach to the central nervous system, the vagus and the splanchnic nerves. The anterior vagal trunk innervates the anterior surface of the stomach almost as far as the pylorus, and the posterior branch innervates the posterior surface except for the distal antrum and pylorus which are innervated by the coeliac branch. The splanchnic nerves follow the blood vessels of the gastric wall. Stimulation of these nerves produces contractions of the stomach. There are two main plexuses of the enteric nervous system, myenteric and submucosal (Figure 4.7). Neurones communicate both with other neurones within the same plexus and the other plexus. They also communicate with sympathetic and parasympathetic branches of the autonomic nervous system. This nervous network regulates the integrated behaviour of the gastrointestinal tract.

The hormonal control of the stomach is an extensive subject and cannot be covered fully here. The amount and time course of the hormone release are affected by the gastric emptying, which, in turn, may be affected by hormone release. Hormone and neural factors together control and optimise the rate of passage of food through the gastrointestinal tract. The major hormones affecting the stomach are secretin, gastrin, cholecystokinin (CCK) and glucose-dependent insulinotropic peptide (GIP). The major stimulus for the release of these hormones is the presence of specific luminal constituents (Table 4.1), although gastrin release is primarily controlled by the vagus.

Table 4.1. - Summary of the actions of the major hormones.

Hormone	Composition & mol. wt. (Daltons)	Local stimuli for release	Major action
Gastrin (G17)	peptide (2117 mw)	peptides, amino	acid secretion
Gastrin (G34)	peptide (3988 mw)	acids, distension	G.I. growth
Secretin	peptide (3056 mw)	duodenal acidity	pancreatic bicarbonate secretion
Cholecystokinin	peptide (3919 mw)	fatty acids amino acids	gallblader contraction pancreatic enzyme secretion and growth
GIP	peptide (5105 mw)	glucose, fatty acids	insulin release

The resting potential, which affects the excitability of the gastric smooth muscle, is about -60 mV and is characterised by rhythmic fluctuations. The oscillations have an amplitude of between 15 and 20 mV and occur approximately every 20 seconds in the stomach. These fluctuations have been termed "slow waves" or "basal electrical rhythm". The rhythmical depolarisation and repolarisation originate from the pacemaker, a group of cells which generate the pacesetter potential. The pacemaker is located on the proximal greater curvature, towards both the lesser curvature and the pyloric region and is the control centre for initiation of peristalsis. Superimposed on the slow waves are small generator potentials, which, when they reach a critical threshold level, give rise to a spike or action potential which produces the contraction of the muscle. Not every pacesetter potential initiates an action potential, since the local threshold value is moderated by neuronal and nervous influences.

Fasted Pattern of Motility
Gastric emptying occurs even during fasting as there is very little absorption of gastric secretion by the gastric mucosa. It is estimated that in the western world 12 to 15 hours per day are spent in the interdigestive phase of motility, with the longest period occurring during sleep. The pattern of electrical activity observed during fasting is markedly different to that observed in the fed state. This activity is called the interdigestive myoelectric cycle or migrating myoelectric complex (MMC) and is often divided into four consecutive phases of activity (Figure 4.8):
Phase 1 - a period of quiescence lasting 40 to 60 minutes with rare contractions

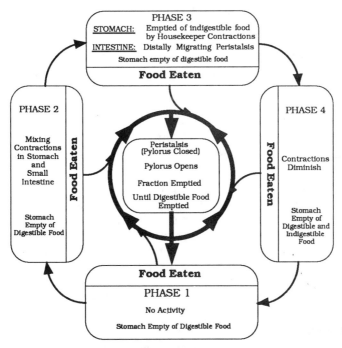

Figure 4.8. - Cycles of gastric motility

Phase 2 - a period of similar duration consisting of intermittent action potentials and contractions that gradually increase in intensity and frequency as the phase progresses. The pressure rises to between 5 and 40 mm Hg during contractions. Phase 3 - a short phase of intense, large regular contractions lasting 4 to 6 minutes. It is the phase which gives the cycle the term the "housekeeper" sequence since it serves to remove from the stomach the large undigested fragments of food. There is a sustained increase in baseline pressure during this phase. When phase three of this cycle reaches the end of the small intestine, phase three of the next cycle is beginning in the duodenum.
Phase 4 - This is a short transitional period between the intense activity of phase 3 and the quiescence of phase 1.

The whole cycle repeats itself every two hours until a meal is ingested, which then immediately initiates the fed patterns of motility.

Effect of food on gastric motility
The empty stomach has a volume of approximately 50 ml which increases to about 1 litre when full. The receptive relaxation of the fundus and upper body is triggered in part by proximal gastric distension and it is effected principally by the inhibitory nerves of the vagus which act on the oblique muscle layer. Stimulation of parasympathetic nerves increases gastric contractility and relaxes the pylorus, resulting in a decrease in the rate of gastric emptying for both solids and liquids. Stimulation of the noradrenergic nerves produces relaxation of the stomach, inhibition of gastric motility and contraction of the pyloric sphincter, also resulting in decreased gastric emptying. The non-adrenergic, non-cholinergic nerves are sometimes referred to as purinergic nerves since stimulation of these nerves with purine bases causes relaxation of gastrointestinal smooth muscle. The exact neurotransmitter for these nerves has not yet been identified.

The stomach empties the three different components of the meal, liquid, digestible solid and indigestible solid, at different rates. A study by Feldman and coworkers (1984) measured the time to half empty the stomach (T50) of 10 oz of a soft drink, scrambled egg and radio-opaque markers (the liquid, digestible solid and indigestible solid phases) as 30 ± 7 minutes, 154 ± 11 minutes and 3 to 4 hours respectively.

The gastric emptying of liquids is not dependent on the activity of the pylorus, but depends on the pressure gradient between pyloric antrum and the duodenum. Thus the slow contractions produced in the proximal stomach which maintain the basal pressure are generally considered to be responsible for the gastric emptying of liquids. The liquid component of a meal empties exponentially, but the emptying of solids is linear after a variable lag time (Figure 4.9).

The antrum is responsible for the breakdown of digestible solids into a suitable size to enable them to pass through the pylorus. During filling of the stomach, the antral contractions are usually weak. The peristaltic waves are soon initiated and they push the contents toward the duodenum. They do not expel food from the stomach, but they cause the larger particles to accumulate away from the walls in a zone where the flow is reversed (Figure 4.10). The larger particles are retropulsed into the antrum, where they are caught up by the next peristaltic wave. Pressures of up to 43 mm Hg have been recorded in the antral mill. The to and fro motion and acid-pepsin digestion accounts for the breakdown of solid food,

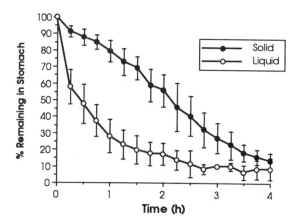

Figure 4.9. - Gastric emptying curves for liquid (lemonade) and digestible solid (scrambled egg) phases of a test meal

while the diameter of the pylorus acts as a sieve retaining large particles for further digestion. Emptying of the pylorus occurs in discrete episodes of 2 to 5 second duration and the majority occur as the terminal antrum, pylorus and duodenum relax at the end of each peristaltic cycle (King *et al.*, 1984).

A transverse mid-gastric band was first noted by William Beaumont in 1833 (republished in 1955) which has subsequently been found to separate the function of proximal and distal stomach. The distribution of food across the proximal and distal band is believed to be a major cause of the lag phase noted when studying the emptying of solids (Moore *et al.*, 1986; Collins *et al.*, 1987). The lag phase is dependent on the size of the food particles in the stomach and the larger the particles, the longer the stomach requires to break them down into a size suitable to exit through the pylorus. Eventually all the digestible material is emptied from

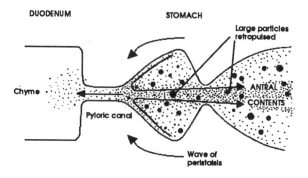

Figure 4.10. - The antral mill demonstrating retropulsion of large solid particles

the stomach into the small intestine where absorption of nutrients occurs, leaving a residue in the stomach of mucus and undigested solids. This includes large particulate matter which cannot pass through the partly closed pylorus. These materials remain in the stomach until the fasted pattern of motility is initiated, which serves to sweep the unwanted material to the ileo-caecal junction.

Factors Influencing Gastric Emptying.

The composition of chyme is the major regulator of gastric emptying. Isocaloric concentrations of fat, carbohydrate and protein leave the stomach at similar rates and the rate of gastric emptying of a meal can be predicted by its nutritive density (Hunt and Stubbs, 1975). Emptying of neutral, isoosmotic, calorifically inert solutions is rapid (Hunt, 1961), but as acidity, osmolarity and calorific value increase, generally the gastric emptying rate slows down (Hunt and Knox, 1972). Studies conducted in our laboratories, to investigate the gastric emptying of meals and its effect in relation to drug absorption, have shown that manipulation of the relative proportions of fat and carbohydrate to formulate meals of identical nutritive density but with different proportions of fat yields similar mean gastric emptying curves.

The inhibitory effect of a fatty acid on gastric emptying may be related to size, as acids with high molecular weight cause less suppression than those of low molecular weight (Hunt and Knox, 1972). Fatty acids, monoglycerides and diglycerides all delay gastric emptying, with a chain length of 14 carbon atoms, myristic acid, giving the most potent effect (Hunt and Knox, 1968). The emptying of amino-acids (except L-tryptophan) is determined by the osmolarity of the solution (Stevens *et al.*, 1975).

Fluids at body temperature leave the stomach more rapidly than fluids which are either warmer or colder, and generally, small volumes of fluid leave the stomach more slowly than large volumes.

Gastric emptying times show considerable variation both between subjects and according to the testing method used. Women have a slower gastric emptying rate then men. The female hormone progesterone increases gastrointestinal transit time and reduces lower oesophageal sphincter tone. Thus, during the luteal phase of the menstrual cycle (days 18-20 of a 28 day cycle) and during pregnancy when progesterone levels are increased, women tend to suffer from gastro-oesophageal reflux and have a delayed gastrointestinal transit (Van Thiel *et al.*, 1977, Wald *et al.*, 1981). Age and obesity have also been found to have a variable effect on the transit of solids and liquids depending on the group of subjects studied and the test method used.

BEHAVIOUR OF PHARMACEUTICAL DOSAGE FORMS

As indicated previously, gastric emptying is the major factor controlling the absorption of all materials entering the body through the oral route. Gastric emptying, pH and motility of the stomach are dependent upon many variables including diet, health and medication, and consequently a thorough knowledge of these factors is useful to allow the optimisation of orally administered formulations. The period for which a dose form remains in the environment of each region of the gastrointestinal tract is determined by local motility patterns.

Gastric Residence Time of Dosage Forms
The major source of variability in the behaviour of dosage forms is the presence of food in the stomach, which produces significant changes in the gastric motility patterns. The rate at which gastric emptying occurs can be a controlling factor in the onset of drug absorption (Heading *et al.*, 1973). The specific effect of food on the behaviour of a particular drug formulation is unpredictable since food can increase, decrease or delay the absorption of a drug. It is convenient to deal with the emptying of the different major types of formulations separately.

Liquids
Gamma scintigraphy has been used to investigate the gastric emptying time of liquid formulations. It has been demonstrated that 10 to 20 ml of a liquid antacid or anti-reflux agent administered to fasted subjects can empty from the stomach within 1 hour (Jenkins *et al.*, 1983; Washington *et al.*, 1986) (Figure 4.11). Gastric residence of the same formulation can be increased to more than 2 hours by the ingestion of a meal 30 minutes prior to administration (May *et al.*, 1984) (Figure 4.12).

Single units as tablets or capsules
Large tablets or capsules, whether intact or in large fragments, will be treated by the stomach as an indigestible material since they do not possess a significant calorific value. The gastric residence time of large units which do not disintegrate within the stomach, given to a fasted individual, can thus be highly variable ranging

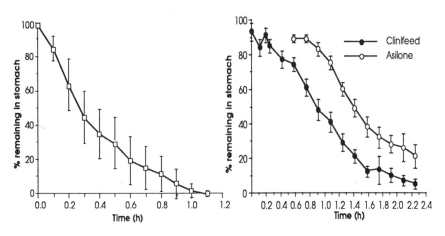

Figure 4.11. - Gastric emptying of 10 ml antacid in fasted volunteers

Figure 4.12. - Gastric emptying of 10 ml antacid (Asilone) given 30 minutes after a meal (Clinifeed)

from 5 minutes to 3 hours, since they rely on the MMC to empty (Kaus *et al.*, 1984; Wilson *et al.*, 1984). A study by Park and co-workers (1984) examined the effect of size and shape of tablets on the rate of their gastric emptying in fasted volunteers. The largest tablet studied was 17.6 x 9.5 mm. It was reported that the physical properties of the tablets did not affect the gastric emptying time and 80% of the dose forms emptied within 2 h.

When large non-disintegrating units are given after a light meal (1500 kJ) the emptying becomes more predictable at around 2 to 3 hours (Wilson *et al.*, 1989). The meal serves to put the motility cycles into phase by initiating fed patterns and the units empty when the first MMC occurs, which is approximately 2 hours after the digestible phase of the meal has emptied. There have been several studies which have demonstrated that large non-disintegrating tablets can remain in the stomach for up to 12 hours if they are administered with a large breakfast (3600 kJ) and if the subject is fed at regular intervals throughout the day (Davis *et al.*, 1984; Wilson *et al.*, 1989). If the tablet is enteric coated, or the drug is not acid soluble, the appearance of the drug in the plasma can be greatly delayed in fed subjects.

Multiparticulate preparations
A popular method of delivering sustained release oral preparations is the multiparticulate or pelleted system contained within a hard gelatin capsule. It would be expected that this method of dosing would overcome the problems of gastric retention in the presence of a meal with a large calorific value. Christensen and coworkers (1985) and Hunter and coworkers (1982) have described the emptying of pellets from fasted subjects as a random event, with the particles tending to empty as a series of boluses. Gruber and coworkers (1987) reported that the pellets empty into the duodenum entrapped in mucus plugs. The emptying of pellets is dependent upon the nature of the capsule and how quickly it disperses, since the volume of fluid available for dissolution is low in the stomach of a fasted individual. The pellets empty more slowly in the presence of food, since they are dispersed in a large volume of meal. The amount of chyme which is delivered to the duodenum is controlled to provide a constant calorific load. This has the effect of delivering the pellets in the meal to the duodenum over a longer period, thus increasing the spread of the pellets over the absorbing surface of the small intestine.

Studies conducted by Meyer and coworkers in dogs (1985a,b) have demonstrated that spheres empty from a food filled stomach as a function of their diameter, their density and the viscosity of the gastric contents. The smaller the diameter (between 1 and 5 mm), the faster the spheres emptied; however, spheres smaller than 1 mm did not empty any faster than 1 mm spheres. Spheres which were more or less dense than water emptied more slowly than the same size spheres with a density of 1. The explanation given is that the lighter spheres floated and the heavier spheres sank and so moved out of the central aqueous stream. Increasing the viscosity of the gastric contents caused even large dense spheres to empty more quickly, possibly because it retarded the layering of the spheres to the base of the stomach. This phenomenon has been observed in human subjects dosed with different density

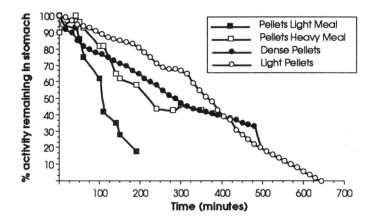

Figure 4.13. - Gastric emptying of different density pellets with various sizes of meals

pellets. Pellets which floated on or sank to the base of the stomach emptied more slowly then pellets of a similar density to food. Even though the light and heavy pellets were administered with a light meal, their emptying was similar to that seen with pellets of a similar density to food when administered with a heavy meal (Figure 4.13). This also indicates that the light and heavy pellets are not caught up in the antral flow.

The discrimination between the emptying of dosage forms produced in the presence of food can clearly be seen when two types of formulations are administered simultaneously. In a study carried out at Nottingham, a large capsule (Osmet®, Alza Corporation, U.S.A) was administered with pellets to subjects after a light or a heavy breakfast in a cross-over study (Figure 4.14). When given with the light breakfast, the Osmet® had emptied by 2 hours amidst the pellets in the majority of subjects; however, the heavy breakfast greatly delayed the gastric emptying of the

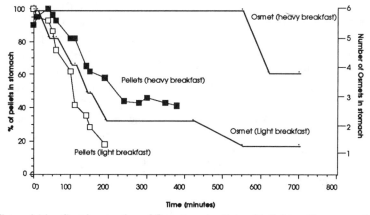

Figure 4.14. - Gastric retention of Osmets and pellets with light and heavy meals

Osmet® to more than 9 hours. The emptying of the pellets was slightly prolonged by the heavier meal (Davis *et al.*, 1984). In general, the pellets emptied as a series of boluses from the stomach, ahead of the tablets which were expelled with the onset of the housekeeper sequence. In some cases the pellet formulations failed to disintegrate, and they too were emptied as a single bolus.

Dispersion of Dose Forms in the Stomach

The most commonly used type of dosage form is the tablet. Endoscopy has demonstrated that when multiple tablets were administered, all lay in the same place in the stomach, at the base of the greater curvature. This is a particular problem with formulations which cause gastric irritation or damage, for example non-steroidal anti-inflammatory drugs which can produce focal erosions due to repeated insult to a small area of the mucosa. Iatrogenically-produced ulcers can be differentiated from those of natural origin, since drug-induced erosions usually occur at the base of the greater curvature, whereas peptic ulcers form on the lesser curvature.

Hard gelatin capsules

Hard gelatin capsules have found a variety of applications in drug formulation. The capsule can be used as a container for powdered drug, multiparticulate systems, a liquid-fill matrix or oily vehicle. The nature of the interior of the fill of the capsule is known to affect the rate of disintegration within the stomach. A hydrophobic interior reduces the rate of disintegration compared to that of a water soluble material, and in addition it reduces the dispersion of the released material. From our own observations and the experiments of Hunter and co-workers (1980, 1982, 1983) it has been established that the dispersion of the capsule fill is limited in fasted subjects and the material empties from the stomach as a bolus. The dispersion is increased if the capsule is taken with a meal, particularly if the meal has a high liquid content. This is of importance since patients are often instructed to take medications with a meal, but it is unclear whether this means before, during or after food.

A recent study in our laboratory has examined the effects of the time of dosing of capsule formulations relative to a standard meal (O'Reilley *et al.*, 1987). The behaviour of a multiparticulate dosage form was followed in six healthy volunteers who received a capsule containing radiolabelled 'Amberlite' resin beads 10 minutes prior to, during and 10 minutes after a meal of a total energy content of 3800 kJ. The particles were released from all capsules within a few minutes. After dosing with the capsule during or after a meal, the pellets tended to remain in the upper half of the stomach. In these cases, the gastric emptying pattern was approximately linear with time (Figure 4.15). The gastric emptying half-times (T50) were similar for all the experiments, being between 3 and 4 hours; however, over the initial 100 minutes, the particles taken before the meal emptied fastest and the emptying followed an exponential pattern with time.

In a second experiment, the gastric emptying of pellets predispersed in a meal was

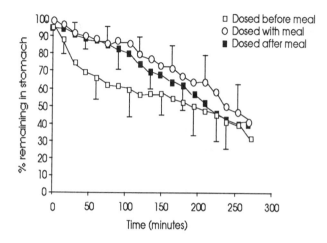

Figure 4.15. - Gastric emptying of pellets dosed immediately before, with or after a meal

compared to that of a capsule containing the same number of pellets. Sprinkling of pellets onto a meal has been suggested for theophylline administration. Although the distribution in the stomach of the predispersed pellets was more uniform, the gastric emptying following both manoeuvres was similar, with no significant differences between the emptying rates (Figure 4.16) (O'Reilley *et al.*, 1987). These systems have two potential drawbacks. Firstly, "sprinkle" systems have to be dispersed into a high viscosity medium, e.g. jam or mashed potatoes, otherwise they may fall through the meal prior to eating, with the consequent risk of under-dosing. Additionally, particles as large as 800 μm are probably unsuit-

able as the subjects complained of the sensation of "grittiness", when eating their meal. This increases the desire to masticate and for sustained release formulations would increase the risk of dose-dumping. Thus it is a prerequisite of such systems that they be relatively small, preferably under 100 μm.

Soft gelatin capsules
There have been relatively fewer studies of the behaviour of soft gelatin capsules in man. From our pilot studies, we have observed that the

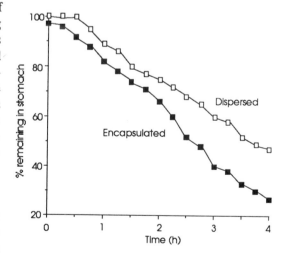

Figure 4.16. - Emptying of pellets dosed in a hard gelatin capsule or sprinkled over a meal

time of disintegration of soft gelatin capsule formulations is highly variable, particularly if the formulations are given without food. The capsules were predominantly broken up as they entered the pylorus immediately prior to leaving the stomach.

A group at the Welsh School of Pharmacy has compared the dispersion of oils from soft gelatin capsules in man and rabbits using x-ray techniques and gamma scintigraphy (Armstrong *et al.*, 1983). Soft gelatin capsules were filled with iodinated cotton seed oil (Lipiodol) for x-ray studies, or iodine-123 labelled ethyl oleate for gamma camera studies in humans. The effects of various surfactants were also investigated. In x-ray studies of rabbits, disintegration of the capsule began after 2 to 3 minutes, swelling into a more isometric shape. This behaviour was observable *in vitro* and was associated with the breakdown of the capsule at the sealing line. Subsequently it was difficult to assess whether the shell had dissolved with the oil as one discrete globule, or whether the oil had emerged from the shell before it had completely dissolved. When a surfactant (1% polysorbate 80) was added to the formulation, the mean disintegration time of the soft gelatin capsule decreased markedly.

Fast dissolving dosage forms
An interesting phenomenon observed in our laboratories concerned with the behaviour of fine particulates in the stomach has recently been reported (Washington *et al.*, 1989). Using a freeze dried formulation base, small fast-dissolving tablets were labelled by inclusion of micronised technetium-99m labelled resin. Gamma scintigraphic studies demonstrated that a radiolabelled micronised Amberlite CG-400 resin delivered in this formulation to fasted volunteers demonstrated a surprising degree of coating of the oesophagus and the stomach (Figure 4.17). This behaviour was noted to contrast with most other dose forms, including liquid and tablet products containing the same marker, which dispersed only in the lower stomach. An explanation for this phenomenon may be that the enhanced dispersion of the micronised resin coupled with the low dosing volume favours stomach retention. Park and Robinson (1984) comment that highly charged polyanions have effective bioadhesive properties and it may therefore be possible that a strongly basic anion exchange resin behaves similarly.

Methods of increasing gastric residence
Gastric Flotation
As will be discussed in Chapter 5, there are few feasible strategies to increase intestinal contact time; however a method of prolonging exposure of the upper small intestine to high concentrations of drug is to retain the drug delivery system in the stomach. This approach is particularly advantageous for acid soluble drugs. The major problem when trying to design a dosage form which has a reproducibly long gastric residence time, or which increases the contact time of a drug with the gastric mucosa, is to overcome the natural function of the stomach which is to act as a temporary store for food. Also the gastric residence time must be unaffected by the large variation which occurs in the food intake of different individuals.

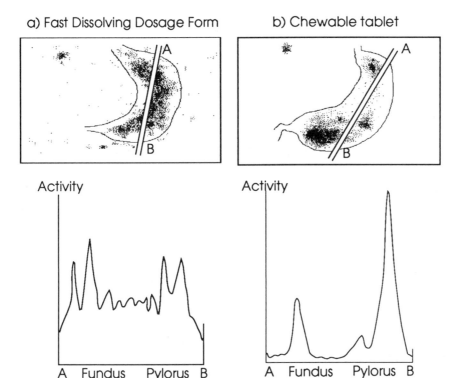

Figure 4.17. - Profile of distribution of activity in the stomach from micronised ion-exchange resin labelled with technetium-99m delivered in a Fast Dissolving Dosage Form and a chewable tablet.

Alginate and hydroxypropylmethylcellulose based tablets have been shown to float on gastric contents and have been used to produce gastric sustained release formulations (Davis *et al.*, 1986; Müller-Lissner *et al.*, 1981; Sheth and Tossounian, 1984). However, it has been concluded by many workers that floating systems do not possess an inherent ability for gastric retention, but rely on the presence of a meal to retard their emptying (Müller-Lissner *et al.*, 1981, Mazer *et al.*, 1988). In addition, the gastric emptying times for both floating and non-floating single units are short in fasted subjects (less than 2 hours), but are prolonged after a meal (around 4 hours) (Müller-Lissner and Blum, 1981; Davis *et al.*, 1986). In the study by Davis and coworkers pellets of different density were also studied. It was demonstrated that initially the heavy pellets emptied from the stomach faster than the light pellets when administered after food. There was, however, no overall difference in gastric emptying or colon arrival times. It was demonstrated in a study by Mazer and coworkers (1988) that the prolonged gastric residence time seen with a floating modified-release formulation of isradipine was not responsible for the slow absorption of the drug, because the majority of the drug release was believed to occur in the colon rather than the stomach.

Floating capsules can be retained in the stomach for prolonged periods as long as food is present in the stomach. In pilot studies for a major pharmaceutical company, a floating capsule was administered to fasted and fed subjects. The fed subjects were allowed food at normal intervals i.e. breakfast, coffee and biscuits at 11 am, lunch etc. The capsules were retained until they broke up in the stomach 12 hours later. In the fasted subjects, the capsules were expelled from the stomach within the first 2 hours of the study.

Patents for floating dosage forms have displayed considerable ingenuity. A patent issued to the Alza Corporation describes a capsule consisting of a balloon containing a volatile liquid such as cyclopentane or ether. The solvent when warmed filled the balloon with vapour, enabling the drug reservoir to float. To enable the unit to exit from the stomach, the device contained a biodegradable plug to allow the vapour to escape. Clearly, this type of dosage form could not be recommended for smokers!

Floating liquid alginate preparations, e.g. Liquid Gaviscon, are used in the treatment of reflux oesophagitis. The formulation consists of a mixture of alginate and sodium bicarbonate, which reacts with gastric acid to form a floating layer on the gastric contents. Although they are not specifically designed to deliver pharmacologically active compounds, their behaviour has been studied in our laboratories in some depth and studies yield important information on the limitations of floating dosage forms, particularly the effect of posture. A study by Bennett and coworkers (1984) demonstrated that an alginate raft emptied faster than food in subjects lying on their left side or their backs and slower in subjects lying on their right side with the raft positioned in the greater curvature. When the subject lay on his left side the raft was presented to the pylorus ahead of the meal and so emptied first.

Anti-reflux preparations, like floating capsules, do not possess an inherent ability to remain in the stomach but require the presence of food to prolong their gastric residence times. For example, half of a 10 ml dose of Liquid Gaviscon had emptied from the stomach of fasted subjects by 20 minutes (T50), but when this dose was given 30 minutes after a test meal of 1693 kJ, the T50 was increased to more than 3 hours. A recent study carried out by our group has shown that an alginate raft can be refloated and its gastric residence time prolonged by small but regular intake of food (Washington, unpublished observation).

Swelling Devices
One approach to increase the gastric residence time of a dosage form is to allow it to swell in the stomach making it too large to pass through the pylorus. A wafer device has been investigated in dogs which is administered as a roll and opens out in the stomach to a square enabling the release characteristics of the drug to be predicted (Figure 4.18). It would be predicted that during fasting, the MMC would still sweep the dosage form out into the small intestine, unless it was extremely large, in which case it would have to be biodegradable. Units made of biodegrad-

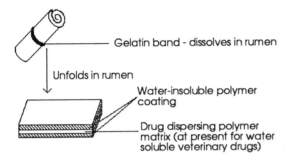

Gelatin band - dissolves in rumen

Unfolds in rumen

Water-insoluble polymer coating

Drug dispersing polymer matrix (at present for water soluble veterinary drugs)

Figure 4.18. - Rolled wafer device for veterinary use

able glass already have a veterinary use, but much work has to be carried out to assess their suitability for human administration.

Materials which can aggregate in the stomach may be retained for long period. Russell and Bass (1985) fed dogs with slurries of polycarbophil particulates (1 to 3 mm in diameter) at doses of 30 and 90 g. The meal containing the 90 g polycarbophil slurry demonstrated a decreased rate of gastric emptying. At autopsy, the particles were shown to have formed large intragastric boluses. The authors proposed that the slow rate of emptying of the polycarbophil was due to the action of the stomach squeezing the particles together, causing a loss of surface-bound water and forming a large bolus.

In a related manner bezoars, accretions of vegetable fibre and mucus, form in animals including man, particularly in patients with abnormal gastric function who have had extensive gastric resection or who are treated with H_2 antagonists. Mucus production is not balanced by degradation in these subjects. Small bezoars are usually passed into the intestine, since the normal stoma (the exit from the stomach) allows the passage of food particles which are 3-4 cm in diameter in the fasted mode. However, small stoma may result in the retention of larger bezoars which have to be removed surgically or treated with enzymes such as raw papain (Rogers *et al.*, 1973).

Bioadhesive Polymers
The use of bioadhesive polymers to provide a localised platform which can adhere to the epithelial surface of the gastrointestinal tract has received extensive study. Early work in the rat showed that the bulk-forming laxative material polycarbophil, a hydrophilic acrylic polymer, adhered to the stomach and intestine. A sustained release formulation containing polycarbophil and albumin was even more effective (Ch'ng *et al.*, 1985; Longer *et al.*, 1985). The proposed mechanism is the formation of hydrogen and electrostatic bonding at the mucus-polymer boundary. Rapid hydration in contact with the muco-epithelial surface appears to favour adhesion, particularly if water can be excluded at the reactive surfaces. Khoshla and Davis (1987) examined the gastric residence of a mixture of technetium-99m labelled Amberlite resin given in a size 0 capsule, together with 100 mg polycarbophil granules. In the small number of subjects studied, no significant effect of the polycarbophil on the retention of pellets was found, although there was not an intimate mixture of polymer and resin.

At the present time it seems that bioadhesion as a mechanism to increase formulation residence in the stomach is not a feasible proposition since the acidic environment and thick mucus blanket prevents association of formulation and polymer. Researchers should regard *in vitro* observations which show association of materials with mucus with caution, since *in vivo* surface mucosal turnover rate is high and bioadhesion for drug delivery can only be utilised if the mucus is still attached to the epithelium.

CONCLUSIONS

The presence or absence of food in the stomach affects the pH, viscosity of the stomach contents, volume of gastric secretion and hence rate of dissolution and degree of spread of the formulation. In addition, it affects the motility patterns, which in the fed state can discriminate between large and small units and in the fasted state emptying can be extremely unpredictable ranging from a few minutes to 3 hours.

The erratic emptying of large tablets, enteric coated units or sustained release matrix tablets in fasted subjects can explain the variability observed in drug-plasma profiles. The rationale for using fasted volunteers in clinical trials has been to decrease variability in the onset of drug absorption, but the fasted dosing regime actually introduces a large source of variation due to unpredictable gastric emptying. It would be far better to administer single units with a light meal of energy value no greater than 1500 kJ, which would have the effect of bringing motility patterns into phase. A further point is that the kinetics of gastric emptying and drug absorption are markedly altered by the size of the meal and these effects may be much larger than small changes in bioavailability induced by different formulations.

REFERENCES

Angus J.A. (1982) Histamine receptors - their classification and role in acid secretion. *Proc. Excerpta Medica; Receptor update*. Geneva p29.

Armstrong N.A., James K.C., Girardin H., Burch A., Davies R.L. and Mitchell G.M. (1983) The dispersion of oils from soft gelatin capsules II. *In vivo* experiments. *Int. J. Pharmaceut. Tech. Prod. Mfr.* 4 10-13.

Beaumont W. (1833) Experiments and observations on the gastric juice and the physiology of digestion. Republished (1955) New York, Dover Publishers Inc.

Bennett C.E., Hardy J.G. and Wilson C.G. (1984) The influence of posture on the gastric emptying of antacid. *Int. J. Pharmaceut.* 21 341-347.

Berglindh T., Helander H.F. and Obrink K.J. (1976) The effect of secretagogues on oxygen consumption, aminopyrine accumulation and morphology of isolated gastric glands. *Acta Physiol. Scand.* 97 401-414.

Bumm R. and Blum A.L. (1987) Lessons from prolonged gastric pH monitoring. *Aliment. Pharmacol. Therap.* 1 518S-526S.

Ch'ng H.S., Park H., Kelly P. and Robinson J.R. (1985) Bioadhesive polymers as platforms for oral controlled drug delivery. II Synthesis and evaluation of some swelling water insoluble bioadhesive polymers. *J. Pharm. Sci.* 74 399-405.

Christensen F.N., Davis S.S., Hardy J.G., Taylor M.J., Whalley D.R and Wilson C.G. (1985) The use of gamma scintigraphy to follow the gastrointestinal transit of pharmaceutical formulations. *J. Pharm. Pharmacol.* **37** 91-95.

Collins P.J., Chatterton B.E. and Horowitz M. (1987) Differential emptying rates of proximal and distal stomach in normal volunteers. *J. Nucl. Med.* **28** 605.

Davis S.S., Hardy J.G., Stockwell A., Taylor M.J., Whalley D.R. and Wilson C.G. (1984) The effect of food on the gastrointestinal transit of pellets and an osmotic device (Osmet). *Int. J. Pharmaceut.* **21** 331-340.

Davis S.S., Stockwell A.F., Taylor M.J., Hardy J.G., Whalley D.R., Wilson C.G., Bechgaard H. and Christensen F.N. (1986) The effect of density on the gastric emptying of single and multiple unit dosage forms. *Pharm. Res* **3** 208-213.

Feldman M., Smith H.J. and Simon T.R. (1984) Gastric emptying of solid radioopaque markers:studies in healthy subjects and diabetic patients. *Gastroenterology* **87** 895-902.

Gruber P., Rubinstein A., Li V.H., Bass P. and Robinson J.R. (1987) Gastric emptying of non-digestible solids in the fasted dog. *J. Pharm. Sci.* **76** 117-122.

Heading R.C., Nimmo J., Prescott L.F. and Tothill P. (1973) The dependence of paracetamol absorption on the rate of gastric emptying. *Br. J. Pharmacol.* **47** 415-421.

Hunt J.N. (1961) The osmotic control of gastric emptying. *Gastroenterology* **41** 49-51.

Hunt J.N. and Knox M.T. (1968) Regulation of Gastric Emptying: *Handbook of Physiology*. Section 6 Alimentary Canal. Ed Code C.F. Baltimore, The Williams and Wilkins Co. 1917-1935.

Hunt J.N. and Knox M.T. (1972) The slowing of gastric emptying by four strong acids and three weak acids. *J. Physiol. (Lond).* **222** 187-208.

Hunt J.N. and Stubbs D.F. (1975) The volume and energy content of meals as determinants of gastric emptying. *J. Physiol. (Lond)* **245** 209-225.

Hunter E., Fell J.T., Calvert R.T. and Sharma H. (1980) *In vivo* disintegration of hard gelatin capsules in fasting and non-fasting subjects. *Int. J. Pharmaceut.* **4** 175-183.

Hunter E., Fell J.T. and Sharma H. (1982) The gastric emptying of pellets contained in hard gelatin capsules. *Drug Devel. Ind. Pharm.* **8** 751-757.

Hunter E., Fell J.T. and Sharma H. (1983) The gastric emptying of hard gelatin capsules. *Int. J. Pharmaceut.* **17** 59-64.

Jenkins J.R.F., Hardy J.G. and Wilson C.G. (1983) Monitoring antacid preparations in the stomach using gamma scintigraphy. *Int. J. Pharmaceut.* **14** 143-148.

Kaus L.C., Fell J.T., Sharma H. and Taylor D.C. (1984) On the intestinal transit of a single non-disintegrating object. *Int. J. Pharmaceut.* **20** 315-323.

Khoshla R. and Davis S.S. (1987) The effect of polycarbophil on the gastric emptying of pellets. *J. Pharm. Pharmacol.* **39** 47-49.

King P.M., Adam R.D., Pryde A., McDicken W.N. and Heading R.C. (1984) Relationships of human antroduodenal motility and transpyloric movement: non-invasive observations with real time ultrasound. *Gut* **25** 1384-1391.

Longer M.A., Ch'ng H.S. and Robinson J.R. (1985) Bioadhesive polymers as platforms for oral controlled drug delivery III: oral delivery of chlorthiazide using a bioadhesive polymer. *J. Pharm. Sci.* **74** 406-411.

May H.A., Wilson C.G. and Hardy J.G. (1984) Monitoring radiolabelled antacid preparations in the stomach. *Int. J. Pharmaceut.* **19** 169-176.

Mazer N., Abisch E., Gfeller J-C., Laplanche R., Bauerfeind P., Cucala M., Lukachich M. and Blum A. (1988) Intragastric behaviour and absorption kinetics of a normal and floating modified-release capsule of isradipine under fasted and fed conditions. *J. Pharm. Sci.* **77** 647-657.

McLaughlan G., Fullarton G.M., Crean G.P. and McColl K.E.L. (1989) Comparison of gastric body and antral pH: a 24 hour ambulatory study in healthy volunteers. *Gut* **30** 573-578.

Meyer J.H., Dressman J., Fink A.S. and Amidon G. (1985a) Effect of size and density on canine gastric emptying of non-digestible solids. *Gastroenterology* **89** 805-813.

Meyer J.H., Gu Y.G., Dressman J. and Amidon G. (1985b) Effect of viscosity and flow rate on gastric emptying of solids (abstract). *Gastroenterology* **88** 1501.

Moore J.G., Dubois A., Christian P.E., Elgin D. and Alazraki N. (1986) Evidence for a midgastric transverse band in humans. *Gastroenterology* **91** 540-545.

Müller-Lissner S.A., Müller-Duysing W., Heinzel F. and Blum A.L. (1981) Floating capsules with slow release of active agents. *Dtsch. Med. Wschr.* **106** 1143-1147.

Müller-Lissner S.A. and Blum A.L. (1981) The effects of specific gravity and eating on gastric emptying of slow release capsules. *New Eng. J. Med.* **304** 1365-1366.

O'Reilly S., Wilson C.G. and Hardy J.G. (1987) The influence of food on gastric emptying of multiparticulate dosage forms. *Int. J. Pharmaceut.* **34** 213-216.

Park H.M., Chernish S.M., Rosenek B.D., Brunelle R.L., Hargrove B. and Wellman H.N. (1984) Gastric emptying of enteric coated tablets. *Dig. Dis. Sci.* **29** 207-212.

Park K. and Robinson J.R. (1984) Bioadhesive polymers as platforms for oral-controlled drug delivery; method to study bioadhesion. *Int. J. Pharmaceut.* **19** 107-127.

Rogers L.F., Davis E.K. and Harle T.S. (1973) Phytobezoar formation and food boli following gastric surgery. *New Engl. J. Med.* **119** 280-290.

Russell J. and Bass P. (1985) Canine gastric emptying of polycarbophil: an indigestible, particulate substance. *Gastroenterology* **89** 307-312.

Sheth P.R. and Tossounian J. (1984) Hydrodynamically balanced system (HBS)™. A novel drug delivery system for oral use. *Drug Dev. Ind. Pharm.* **10** 313-339.

Stevens J.R., Woolson R.F. and Cooke A.R. (1975) Effects of essential and non-essential amino acids on gastric emptying in the dog. *Gastroenterology* **69** 920-927.

Van Thiel D.H., Gavaler J.S., Joshi S.N., Sara R.K. and Stremple J. (1977) Heartburn in pregnancy. *Gastroenterology* **72** 666-668.

Wald A., Van Thiel D.H., Hoechstetter L., Gaveler J.S., Egler K.M., Verm R., Scott L. and Lester R. (1981) Gastrointestinal transit: the effect of the menstrual cycle. *Gastroenterology* **80** 1497-1500.

Washington N., Washington C. and Wilson C.G. (1986) The effect of food on the gastric emptying of a floating alginate raft. Society for Drug Research, Cambridge.

Washington N., Wilson C.G., Greaves J.L., Norman S., Peach J.M. and Pugh K. (1989) A gamma scintigraphic study of gastric coating by Expidet, tablet and liquid formulations. *Int. J. Pharmaceut.* (in press).

Wilson C.G., Parr G.D., Kennerley J.W., Taylor M.J., Davis S.S., Hardy J.G. and Rees J.G. (1984) Pharmacokinetics and *in vivo* scintigraphic monitoring of a sustained release acetylsalicylic acid formulation. *Int. J. Pharmaceut.* **18** 1-8.

Wilson C.G., Washington N., Greaves J.L., Kamali F., Rees J.A., Sempik A.K. and Lampard J.F. (1989) Bimodal release of ibuprofen in a sustained-release formulation: a scintigraphic and pharmacokinetic open study in healthy volunteers under different conditions of food intake. *Int. J. Pharmaceut.* **50** 155-161.

5

Small intestine: transit and absorption of drugs

The small intestine is between 5 and 6 metres in length and its main functions are to mix food with enzymes to facilitate digestion, circulate the intestinal contents with the intestinal secretions to enable absorption to occur and propel the unabsorbed materials in an aboral direction. This tissue has the highest capacity for nutrient and drug absorption within the gastrointestinal tract due to the large surface area provided by epithelial folding and the villous structures of the absorptive cells.

ANATOMY AND PHYSIOLOGY OF THE SMALL INTESTINE
Gross Morphology
The small bowel is arbitrarily divided into three parts, the first 20 to 30 cm is termed the duodenum, the second 2.5 metres the jejunum and the final 3.5 metres the ileum. These regions are not anatomically distinct, although there are differences in absorptive capability and secretion. There is no definite sphincter between the stomach and duodenum although in some studies a zone of elevated pressure between the two regions has been reported to exist. The duodenum has a thick wall with a deeply folded mucous membrane and contains duodenal digestive glands and Brunner's glands. Brunner's glands are found only in the submucosa of the duodenum. They produce a protective alkaline secretion which neutralizes gastric acid and does not contain any enzymes. The jejunum is thicker walled and more vascular than the duodenum and has larger and more numerous villi than the ileum. In the ileum, the lymphatic follicles (Peyer's patches) are larger and more numerous than elsewhere in the intestine.

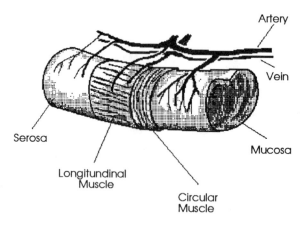

Figure 5.1. - Section of the small intestine

Mucosa
The small intestine consists of the serosa, the muscularis, the submucosa and the mucosa (Figure 5.1). The serosa is an extension of the peritoneum, and consists of a single layer of flattened mesothelial cells overlying some loose connective tissue. The muscularis has an outer longitudinal layer and an inner circular layer of muscle. The submucosa consists largely of dense connective tissue sparsely infiltrated by lymphocytes, fibroblasts, macrophages, eosinophils, mast and plasma cells. The submucosa contains an extensive lymphatic network.

The intestinal mucosa itself can be divided into three layers:
a) the *muscularis mucosa* which is the deepest layer consisting of a sheet of muscle 3 to 10 cells thick that separates the mucosa from the submucosa.
b) the *lamina propria*, the middle layer, is mainly connective tissue and forms the core of the numerous villi and surrounds the crypts. The *lamina propria* usually contains many types of cells e.g. plasma cells, lymphocytes, mast cells, macrophages, smooth muscle cells and non-cellular elements such as collagen and elastin fibres. The *lamina propria* provides structural support, and there is increasing evidence that it has an important role in preventing the entry of micro-organisms and foreign substances.
c) the epithelium is the innermost layer of the mucosa. It consists of a single layer of columnar epithelial cells or enterocytes, which line both the crypts and the villi.

Crypts
The cells between the villi form the germinal area known as the crypts. The main functions of the crypts are cell renewal, water, ion, exocrine and endocrine secretion. The crypt epithelium consists of at least 4 different cell types:
a) *the Paneth cells* which secrete large amounts of protein-rich materials and in the rat are known to phagocytose selected protozoa and bacteria. Human Paneth cells contain lysozyme, IgA and IgG.
b) *goblet cells* which secrete mucus. These cells are able to tolerate a higher osmotic stress than the enterocytes and are more firmly attached to the basement membrane. Exposure to toxins or hypertonic vehicles leads to accumulation of goblet cells at the apex of the villus, goblet cell capping, and a hypersecretion of mucus presumably as a protective response (Bryan *et al.*, 1980).

c) _undifferentiated cells,_ the most common type, whose major function is in the renewal process of the epithelium.

d) _endocrine cells_ which produce hormones and peptides such as gastrin, secretin, cholecystokinin, somatostatin, enteroglucagon, motilin, neurotensin, gastric inhibitory peptide, vasoactive peptide and serotonin.

The volume of intestinal secretions formed by the cells in the crypts is around 1800 ml per day and is almost pure extracellular fluid, with a pH of between 7.5 and 8.0. The fluid is rapidly absorbed by the villi and provides the watery vehicle required for the absorption of substances from chyme.

Epithelium
The epithelium which covers the intestinal villi is composed of absorptive cells, goblet cells, a few endocrine cells and tuft or calveolated cells. The goblet and endocrine cells closely resemble those found in the crypts. The tuft or calveolated cells are characterized by long, broad apical microvilli and an intra-cytoplasmic system of tubules and vesicles. These cells are uncommon and their function is not known. The absorptive cells or enterocytes are tall, columnar cells, with their nuclei located close to their base.

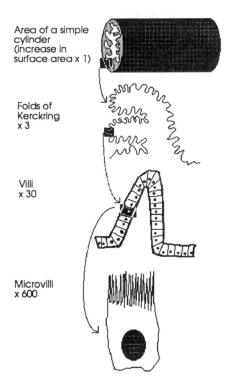

Area of a simple cylinder (increase in surface area x 1)

Folds of Kerckring x 3

Villi x 30

Microvilli x 600

Figure 5.2.- Increase in surface area due to folding, villi and microvilli

Organisation of the Mucosa
The mucosa of the small intestine has a surface area which is greatly increased by the folds of Kerckring, villi and microvilli (brush border) and is about 200 m^2 in an adult (Figure 5.2).

Folds of Kerckring
A particularly prominent feature in the small intestine is the folding of the epithelium, known as the folds of Kerckring. The folds increase the surface area by a factor of 3. These folds extend circularly most of the way around the intestine and and are especially well developed in the duodenum and jejunum, where they protrude by up to 8 mm into the lumen.

Villi
The surface of the mucous membrane of the small intestine possesses about 5 million villi, each about 0.5 to 1 mm long. Although the villi are often described as "finger-like", their shape

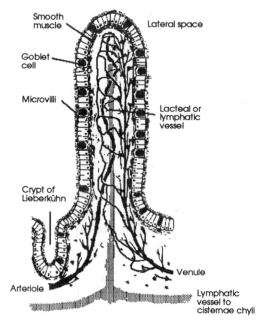

Figure 5.3. - Structure of a villus

changes along the gut and duo-denal villi are shorter and broader than those found in the jejunum. Further down the gut the villus height decreases. Diet and environment markedly affect mucosal morphology and intestinal biopsies demonstrate differences between human populations. There is also a species difference, for example, the villi of the chick are pointed and leaf-like.

The major features of a villus are illustrated in Figure 5.3. Each villus contains an arteri-ole and a venule and also a blind-ending lymphatic vessel called the lacteal. The arteriole and venule do not anastomose in the small intestine as they do in the gastric mucosa. Small molecules absorbed through the villus pass into the descending loop of the villus capillary and diffuse into the ascending vessel. This creates a counter-current exchange system in each villus, which is relatively inefficient since it decreases the concentration gradient for passive diffusion. The efficiency of this process has been estimated to be around 15% (Figure 5.4) and has the net effect of slowing the rate of absorption.

Microvilli

Each enterocyte has about 1000 minute processes or microvilli which project into the intestinal lumen. Multiple actin filaments extending into the interior of each microvillus are believed to be responsible for contraction of the micro-villi and thus movement of the fluid immediately in contact with the surface.

The membrane which forms the micro-villi on the outer surface of the absorptive cells is rich in protein, cholesterol and glycolipids and contains enzymes,

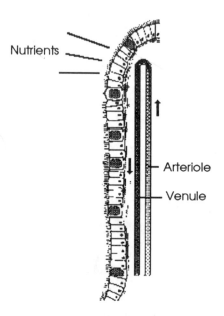

Figure 5.4. - Villus blood flow

disaccharidases and peptidases which are localised within the surface membrane. Specific receptor proteins are located on the microvillus membrane-surface coat complex which selectively bind substances prior to their absorption, including the intrinsic factor-vitamin B12 complex in the ileum and conjugated bile salts in the distal intestine.

The Gastrointestinal Circulation

The gastrointestinal circulation is the largest systemic regional vasculature and nearly one third of the cardiac output flows through the gastrointestinal viscera, with 10% (500 ml min^{-1}) supplying the small intestine. Anatomically, each region, i.e. salivary glands, pharynx, oesophagus, stomach, liver and intestine, possesses separate blood vessels. The blood vessels of the jejunum and ileum are derived from the superior mesenteric artery. Arterioles branch off and supply the muscular coat and form plexuses in the submucosal layer. From each plexus, tiny vessels direct blood to the villi and the glands in the mucosa.

The distribution of the blood flow varies according to the metabolic demands of the cells within each region. The highly metabolic villi receive 60% of the blood flow to the mucous layer, while the muscle layer with it's lower demand for oxygen receives only 20% of the blood flow. During periods of enhanced absorption or electrolyte secretion, the blood flow is preferentially distributed to the mucosa, whilst increased intestinal motility causes diversion of the blood flow to the muscle layers. After a meal, blood flow increases by 30 to 130% of basal flow and the hyperaemia is confined to the segment of the intestine exposed to the chyme. Long chain fatty acids and glucose are the major stimuli for hyperaemia, which is probably mediated by hormones such as cholecystokinin released from mucosal endocrine cells (Granger *et al.*, 1985).

The blood from the small intestine flows into the large hepatic portal vein which takes the blood to the liver. The liver has the highest drug metabolising capacity in the body and, in a single pass, can remove a large proportion of the absorbed drug before it reaches the systemic circulation. This process, termed first-pass metabolism, may have a significant effect on drug bioavailability when formulations are given by the oral route. The blood supply from the buccal cavity and the anal sphincter do not drain to the portal vein and a greater proportion of a drug with a high hepatic extraction may be absorbed from these regions.

THE LYMPHATIC SYSTEM

The lymphatic system is important in the absorption of nutrients, especially fat, from the gastrointestinal tract and provides a route by which electrolytes, protein and fluids can be returned from the interstitial spaces to the blood. It is also responsible for removal of red blood cells lost into tissues as a result of haemorrhage or bacteria which may have invaded tissues.

Structure of the Lymphatics

The gastrointestinal tract is richly supplied with lymphatic vessels. Lymphatic

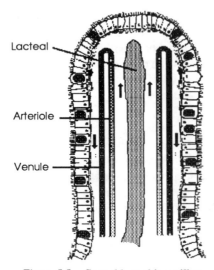

Lacteal

Arteriole

Venule

Figure 5.5. - Central lacteal in a villus

vessels are lined by flattened endothelium with an incomplete basement membrane. The larger lymph vessels also are surrounded by smooth muscle and connective tissue. Contractile activity of lymphatic vessels is most likely to be related to the amount of smooth muscle associated with it. The valves found in the larger vessels assist with the propulsion of lymph.

In the oesophagus, stomach and intestine, there is a plexus of lymph vessels present in the mucosal, submucosal and muscular layers with short vessels linking the networks together passing through lymph nodes which act as filters for lymph directed into larger vessels. The major lymphatic trunks are found on the left side of the body with the bulk of the lymph entering the circulation at the left jugulo sub-clavian tap which is at the base of the neck.

The lymphatic vessels of the small intestine are called the lacteals (Figure 5.5). The central lymphatic vessel is a blind-ending tube. The walls consist of a single layer of thin endothelium and resemble blood capillaries, however, the small fenestrations seen in the blood vessel walls are not found in the lymphatics. The intestinal villi rhythmically contract and relax which probably serves to pump lymph into the lacteals of the submucosa. The flow of lymph in the thoracic duct is about 1-2 ml min^{-1} between meals but this can increase by 5 to 10 fold during absorption and digestion of a meal.

Lymphatic tissue can also be found in certain areas of the gastrointestinal tract close to epithelial surfaces or as large aggregates e.g. pharyngeal tonsils and Peyer's patches in the ileum. The lymphoid tissue of Peyer's patches is usually situated on the ante-mesenteric border. Each patch typically comprises of 40 to 50 nodules which are separated from the gut lumen by a layer of epithelial cells, the M-cells. There is a thin layer of vascularised connective tissue between the nodules and the serosa. The patches have their own blood supply. M-cells lack fully developed microvilli, are pinocytic and contain numerous vesicles. These cells may play a key role in the intestinal immune response since they transport macromolecules and therefore have a specific role in antigen uptake. At this point in the intestine the mucosal barrier may be breached by pathogens.

Formation of Lymph
Lymph is a component of the extracellular fluid of the body and is largely derived from fluid and solute filtered from the blood circulation across the capillary wall. The fluid content of the blood is controlled by a mixture of hydrostatic forces and

osmotic pressure. The high pressure within the arteriolar capillaries forces plasma into the intercellular spaces, the majority of which is returned to the bloodstream at the venous end of the capillary. The volume and solute concentration of the filtrate is modified by passage through the tissues and the lymphatic vessel endothelium before becoming lymph. About 10% of the fluid flowing from the arterial capillaries is absorbed by the lymphatic capillaries and returns to the bloodstream through the lymphatic system.

The sparse and incomplete basement membrane of the endothelium of small lymphatics is a weak barrier to the passage of solutes, fluids and large particles. In addition, the intercellular adhesion is poor and hence large particulates and even cells can occasionally pass between them. Specific vesicular transport may also be an important route of entry.

Composition of Lymph
All plasma proteins are found in lymph. The protein concentration of lymph from all parts of the alimentary tract tends to be high; e.g. thoracic duct lymph has a protein concentration of 66% of that of serum. Lymph contains relatively less of the larger proteins compared to plasma, suggesting that molecular size is important in lymph filtration. Materials with a molecular weight of less than 10,000 are found in similar concentrations in both lymph and plasma. Additional proteins, mainly immunoglobulins, are added to the lymph on passage through the lymph nodes. Finally, lymph also contains reticulo-endothelial cells (lymphocytes) to destroy bacteria.

Lymph contains all the coagulation factors found in the blood, but it clots less readily. The electrolyte composition is very similar. Cholesterol and phospholipids in lymph are mainly associated with protein as lipoprotein and together with triglycerides synthesised in the enterocytes form structures known as chylomicrons. This renders the triglycerides water-miscible. The concentration of chylomicrons varies with the amount of protein present in the lymph. The amount of neutral fat in the chylomicrons depends upon the degree of absorption from the gastrointestinal tract. Immediately after meals there are large quantities of lipoproteins and fats in the lymph which have been taken up from the gastrointestinal tract, but this drops to a low level between meals.

Stimulation of Lymphatic Transport
Many substances given by mouth increase the flow of lymph, e.g. olive oil and corn oil (Yoffey and Cortice, 1970; Tasker, 1951; Borgström and Laurell, 1953). Simmonds (1954) found enhanced flow of lymph in rats after intragastric administration of substances such as water, 0.9% sodium chloride, 10% serum albumin or 10% glucose. Of these, sodium chloride is a particularly potent lymphagogue, and some workers use an intragastric infusion of this solution to maintain a good mesenteric lymph flow in a period immediately after creating a lymph fistula.

SECRETIONS INTO THE SMALL INTESTINE
Glands
Two types of glands are found in the small intestine:
1. Brunner's glands which are confined to the duodenum and secrete bicarbonate and mucus.
2. The intestinal cells, which are present throughout the small intestinal and secrete mucus and a few enzymes.

The intestinal juice or *succus entericus* produced by the intestinal glands has an electrolyte composition similar to that of extracellular fluid. It has a pH of 7.5 to 8.0 and the only enzyme of importance in the *succus entericus* is enteropeptidase (enterokinase), derived from the microvillous membrane, which converts trypsinogen to trypsin.

Pancreatic Secretion
The human pancreas is a large gland, often more than 20 cm long and secretes approximately 1 litre of pancreatic juice per day. The pancreatic juice has two major components:(i) alkaline fluid and (ii) enzymes At all rates of secretion pancreatic juice is isotonic with extracellular fluid. The pancreatic acinar cells synthesize and secrete the majority of the enzymes which digest food. All the pancreatic proteases are secreted as inactive enzyme precursors and are converted to the active form in the lumen whereas pancreatic amylase and lipase are secreted in active forms. The secretion of the aqueous phase and the bicarbonate component is largely regulated by the pH of the chyme delivered into the small intestine from the stomach. The secretion of pancreatic enzymes is primarily regulated by the amount of fat and protein entering the duodenum.

Biliary Secretion
Bile is secreted by the liver. All hepatic cells continually form a small amount of bile which is secreted into bile canaliculi which collects and is concentrated in the gall bladder in man. Concentration takes place by removal of sodium ions, chloride and water then follow.

Bile is a variable and complex mixture of water, organic and inorganic solutes. The daily output is 700 to 1200 ml. The major organic solutes are bile acids, phospholipids (particularly lecithin), cholesterol and bilirubin. Sodium and potassium ions are found in proportions similar to that found in plasma whilst the concentrations of Cl^- and HCO_3^- are often lower and the bile acids make up the remainder of the ion balance.

Bile salts are water-soluble derivatives of cholesterol. Cholic acid and chenodeoxycholic (chenic) acid are synthesized by the liver. Bile acids are poorly absorbed in the proximal small intestine, unlike the majority of nutrients, but are absorbed by an active process in the terminal ileum. After absorption, bile acids have a high hepatic clearance and are re-secreted in the bile. This process is known as enterohepatic recirculation.

Bile salts have two important actions:
(i) emulsification of the fat content of food, by decreasing the surface tension and hence producing small droplets of fat in aqueous suspension.
(ii) assisting in the absorption of fatty acids, monoglycerides, cholesterol and other lipids from the intestinal tract by forming submicron clusters of fat and surfactant called *micelles*.

The major pigment of bile is bilirubin. Its formation is of considerable biological significance as it is the most important means by which haem, produced by the breakdown of haemoglobin, is eliminated. Up to 20% of the bilirubin present in bile is produced from other resources such as myoglobin and cytochromes.

INTESTINAL pH
Gastric pH has been relatively well defined since the stomach is accessible using a Ryle's tube, but fewer studies have investigated intestinal conditions. Data obtained using pH telemetry capsules indicate that the lumen of the proximal jejunum usually lies within the pH range 5.0 to 6.5 rising slowly along the length of the small intestine to reach pH 6 to 7, although high values in the range 7 to 9 have occasionally been found (Hardy *et al.*, 1987).

DIGESTION AND ABSORPTION OF NUTRIENTS
Food assimilation takes place primarily in the small intestine and is optimised by the increased surface area produced by Kerkring's folds, villi and microvilli. The chyme presented to the duodenum from the stomach consists of a mixture of coarsely emulsified fat, protein and some metabolites produced by the action of pepsin, and carbohydrates including starch, the majority of which would have escaped the action of the salivary amylase.

The chyme is acidic and this is buffered by bile and the bicarbonate present in the pancreatic juice to between pH 6.5 and 7.6. Electrolytes and water pass continuously across the small intestine and when there is a net accumulation of fluid in the intestine, secretion is said to have occurred. Secretion occurs under the influences of the hormones glucagon and gastrin but can be stimulated by bacteria. The digestive enzymes are located in the brush border of the glycocalyx and they can be altered by changes in diet, especially by the proportion of ingested disaccharides. The protein content of the diet does not affect the proteases, but a diet deficient in protein leads to a reduction in all enzymes.

Blood passing through the minute veins of the capillaries is brought into close proximity with the intestinal contents in an area estimated to be about 10 m². The capillaries are fenestrated, hence allowing a very rapid exchange of absorbed materials. During digestion and absorption the villi contract fairly quickly at regular intervals and relax slowly. The contraction probably serves to pump lymph into the lacteals of the submucosa and stir the intestinal contents. The veins in the villi ultimately open into the portal vein, which leads directly to the liver and hence all materials carried from the small intestine undergo "first-pass" metabolism.

The site of absorption of the small intestine depends upon the relationship between the rate of transit with that of absorption. This is more apparent for drugs than for food, since excipients may control the rate of drug release. For example the duodenum can be demonstrated to have a high rate of absorption, however, the passage through this region is extremely rapid and the net absorption in this region is probably quite low. The function of the duodenum is to sample the chyme which is delivered from the stomach and thus regulate the delivery of the food according to its calorific value by a feedback process.

Carbohydrates

The principal dietary carbohydrates are starches, sucrose and lactose. Starch is a glucose containing polysaccharide with a molecular weight from 100,000 to more than 1 million Daltons. The two major polysaccharides of starch are amylose and amylopectin. Indigestible carbohydrates, e.g. cellulose, are the main constituents of dietary fibre.

Salivary and pancreatic amylases initiate the hydrolysis of starch and exhibit their optimal activity at near neutral pH. The salivary amylase is inactivated once it reaches the acid in the stomach. The intraluminal digestion of carbohydrates occurs rapidly in the duodenum due to the large amount of amylase secreted by the pancreas. The final oligosaccharide products of luminal digestion are formed before the chyme reaches the jejunum. The major products of starch digestion are maltose and maltotriose. Carbohydrates are absorbed in the proximal part of the small intestine and they have completely disappeared from the lumen by the time the meal reaches the ileum.

The disaccharides are further digested to monosaccharides by the brush border enzymes lactase, sucrase, maltase and isomaltase during their transfer across the epithelium. It is likely that the enzymes and carriers are so orientated spatially that hydrolysis and and subsequent absorption are sequential events. Glucose is absorbed rapidly and completely by both passive diffusion and active transport. The brush border possesses a sodium-dependent carrier which transports sugars across the membrane in either direction.

Proteins

Most protein digestion occurs principally in the small intestine under the influence of the proteolytic enzymes of the pancreatic secretion. When the proteins leave the stomach they are mainly in the form of large polypeptides. Immediately upon entering the small intestine, the partial breakdown products are attacked by the pancreatic enzymes. Trypsin and chymotrypsin split protein molecules into small polypeptides, carboxypolypeptidase then cleaves individual amino acids from the carboxyl ends of the polypeptides. The brush border of the small intestine contains several different enzymes for hydrolysing the remaining small peptides. The constituent amino acids are then absorbed. Most naturally occurring amino acids are L-isomers which are transported against concentration gradients by sodium-dependent carrier mechanisms. There are four carrier systems for amino acids: for neutral amino acids (histidine), for basic amino acids (lysine), for dicarboxylic acids (glutamic acid) and a fourth transports the amino acids proline, hydroxyproline and glycine.

Studies suggest that very small amounts of proteins may be absorbed intact. This is most clearly seen in neonates, where dietary proteins or bacterial exotoxins may either provoke an immune response or confer passive immunity to the host after absorption.

Fats
Dietary intake of lipid is mainly in the form of triglycerides which are composed of a glycerol chain and three fatty acids. There are also small quantities of cholesterol, phospholipids and cholesterol esters in chyme. Fat is emulsified by the bile salts into small droplets which disperse in water allowing access of digestive enzymes.

Lipase in the pancreatic juice and enteric lipase from the epithelial cells of the small intestine both hydrolyse emulsified triglycerides to monoglycerides and fatty acids. The short and medium chain fatty acids are absorbed passively through the epithelium into the blood. The long chain fatty acids and monoglycerides remain as micelles and are internalized by the epithelium. They are reassembled into triglycerides within the cell and excreted into the lymph as small (0.1 μm) droplets called chylomicrons (Figure 5.6).

ABSORPTION OF DRUGS
The principal permeability barrier is represented by the luminal surface of the brush border. Most drugs are absorbed by passive diffusion in their unionised state. The pH of the small intestine determines the degree of ionisation and hence controls the efficiency of absorption; this is the basis of the pH-partition theory of drug absorption which is discussed in Chapter 1. Protein binding at the serosal side of

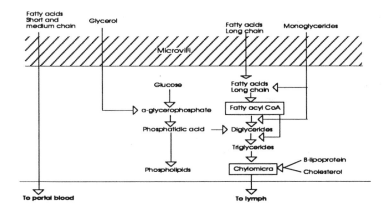

Figure 5.6. - Metabolism and transport of fat into the lymphatic and systemic circulations

the epithelium helps maintain a concentration gradient by binding the absorbed drug, which is then removed by blood flow from the absorption site.

The luminal pH is approximately 7, which suggests that some acidic drugs, such as salicylate, should not be well absorbed. To account for the absorption of these materials is has been proposed that a microclimate exists close to the brush border and the pH is as low as 5.3 (Lucas, 1984). This is supported by microelectrode measurements which suggest a surface pH of between 4.5 and 6.0 which is dependent on the luminal glucose concentration. Unfortunately, this hypothesis suggests that basic drugs would be poorly absorbed, which is not the case. Bases may be absorbed in an ionised form through the paracellular route or they may interact with organic cations which have been found to be secreted from the blood into the lumen of the intestine.

Solvent Drag and Intestinal Permeability

The intestine absorbs approximately 10 litres of water a day from the diet and digestive secretions, and only 100-200 ml of water is lost in the stools. The question of whether the water flux influences drug absorption has been raised by many authors. Kitizawa and co-workers (1975) perfused the rat intestine *in situ* with solutions of varying tonicity and studied the disappearance from the lumen of sulphanilamide, sulphisoxazole and metoclopramide. The disappearance of the drugs was increased with increasing fluid absorption and decreased when the tonicity of the perfusate was increased to cause intestinal secretion. Ochensfahrt and Winne (1974a,b) carried out a similar experiment but measured the appearance in the mesenteric blood of both acidic (benzoic, salicylic) and basic drugs (amidopyrine, antipyrine). The absorption of both types of drugs increased as the water absorption increased. These experiments suggest that increasing water absorption assists drug absorption, a phenomenon known as solvent drag.

Intestinal reserve length

Ho and coworkers (1983) modelled the absorption of drugs in the small intestine using a simple first-order model, which led to the prediction of an exponential decrease in drug concentration with length of small intestine. The authors then derived an index for the potential absorption of compounds based on the distance over which 95% of drug would be absorbed. The length of intestine available over and above this was called the 'intestinal reserve length'. This cannot be applied to certain drugs which are incompletely absorbed; for example the beta-blocker atenolol which is absorbed for 3-4 hours following administration. Absorption then stops abruptly, even though 50% of the dose remains unabsorbed, presumably on entry of the drug into the colon, where it is not absorbed. Similarly hydrochlorothiazide is poorly absorbed in the colon (Taylor, 1989) and hence absorption stops abruptly as the bolus enters this region.

Although intestinal reserve length is a useful guideline, it makes a number of physiological assumptions, primarily that there is no variation in the absorptive capacity of the small intestine along its length. This assumption may be true for some materials, but in other cases absorption may be carrier-mediated or occur at specific sites. In spite of these shortcomings, the model does provide an explanation of a number of phenomena, notably the variation in absorption with transit velocity.

Interaction with Food

The presence of food may influence the absorption of several drugs and can either enhance, delay or reduce absorption (Toothaker and Welling, 1980). Food can adsorb or absorb drug, the metal ions present in food such as milk can chelate drug or the drug can bind to dietary proteins thus changing its bioavailability. The presence of viscous chyme can act as a physical barrier reducing drug access to the absorbing surface.

The absorption of drugs such as penicillin V and G, theophylline and erythromycin is reduced by the presence of food, but food delays absorption of such drugs as cimetidine, metronidazole and digoxin. The effect of food on drug absorption can be dependent on the type of dosage form used, the excipients and the form of the drug, for example erythromycin stearate in film coated tablets demonstrated reduced absorption with food, erythromycin estolate in suspension was unaffected by food but absorption of erythromycin ethylsuccinate in suspension and erythromycin estolate in capsules was increased by the presence of food (Toothaker and Welling, 1980).

Certain components of food, notably fibre, have a particularly important effect on drug absorption. Fibre is known to inhibit the absorption of digoxin and entrap steroids. It is well accepted that foods with a high content of polyvalent metals such as calcium, magnesium, iron, aluminium and zinc, such as milk products, inhibit the absorption of tetracycline and reduce availability. Doxycycline has a slightly lesser tendency to form chelates, thus milk reduces its bioavailability somewhat less than other tetracyclines.

Availability of many drugs is determined by their solubility at the local pH. In the stomach this is highly variable, depending on the presence of food, but the small intestine has a relatively constant pH around 7.0. Drug absorption may be modulated by the presence of food which alters the gastric pH, the viscosity and the transit time through various sections of the gut and a single clear effect may not be evident.

PATTERNS OF MOTILITY IN THE SMALL INTESTINE

The small intestine, like the stomach, displays two distinct patterns of motility. The fed pattern is characterized by random motor activity, in groups of 1 to 3 sequential contractions, separated by 5 to 40 seconds of inactivity. The physical and chemical nature of the food determines the number of contractions; for example, twice as many contractions occur when solid food is ingested than when an equicalorific liquid is consumed (Granger et al., 1985). Carbohydrates stimulate the largest number of contractions, followed by proteins and lipids. The fed pattern of motility consists of segmental and peristaltic contractions, the segmental contractions being

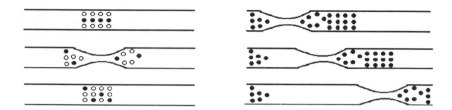

Figure 5.7. - Segmental contractions (left) and propulsive contractions (right) of
the small intestine

the most frequent (Figure 5.7). Initially a segment of the bowel, less than 2 cm in length, contracts while the adjacent segments are relaxed; the procedure is then reversed, as the contracted segment relaxes and vice versa. This type of motility mixes chyme by continually moving it in the lumen and increasing contact with the absorbing surface, but since there are less frequent contractions aborally than orally, there is a net movement of chyme towards the large bowel. This movement is enhanced by peristaltic contractions which occur less frequently than segmental contractions and each move the chyme a few centimetres. The continuous movement shears the chyme resulting in effective mixing (Figure 5.8).

The interdigestive migrating myoelectric complex continues from the stomach to the small intestine. Phase I is a period of no activity, Phase II is characterized by random activity and Phase III is a period of intense activity which is associated with the aboral movement of the intestinal contents. The IMMC occurs every 140 to 150 minutes, and as one complex reaches the ileum, another starts at the duodenum. The velocity of the contractile wave decreases as it approaches the ileum and only rarely does it reach the terminal ileum (Kellow *et al.*, 1986).

Stagnation at the Ileocaecal Junction.
The ileocaecal junction divides the terminal small intestine from the caecum. The junction or sphincter appears to formed by papillary protrusions into the lumen of

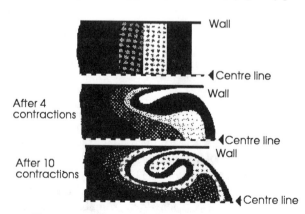

After 4 contractions

After 10 contractions

Figure 5.8. - Laminar mixing produced by repetitive
longitudinal contractions

the caecum, rather than two flat lips of a valve (Phillips, 1989). Its function seems to be to retain chyme in the small intestine until digestion is largely complete and then to empty its contents into the large bowel. The ileocaecal junction also serves to prevent the spread of the colonic bacteria into the small intestine

(Phillips, 1983). Contraction of the ileocolonic sphincter is produced by α-adrenergic agonists including phenylephrine, adrenaline and noradrenaline, and by cholinergic agonists such as bethanechol, whereas pure beta-adrenergic agonists, such as isoprenaline, cause relaxation (Pahlin, 1975).

Scintigraphy often demonstrates accumulation or bunching of material at the ileocaecal junction, followed by spreading of material through the ascending colon. Non-disintegrating matrices may remain at this location for some time; Marvola and co-workers (1987) have reported times ranging from 2 to 20 hours in the ileocaecal region, which agrees with our own observations in young and elderly volunteers (Davis, 1989).

METHODS OF MEASUREMENT OF SMALL INTESTINAL TRANSIT TIME

It has been realised that the time available for drug absorption is a function of the contact time with the small intestine. However, many older textbooks use measurements based on barium X-ray contrast, or indirect methods such as the hydrogen breath test, quote much longer small intestinal transit times than direct measurement with gamma scintigraphy. Barium is not a good model of intestinal contents, and measurements of transit from patients with some form of organic disease, such as those with ileostomies, should be treated with caution.

Two dimensional gamma scintigraphy can be used to measure stomach to caecum transit times, but cannot be used to measure the distance travelled by a unit through segments of the small intestine since it is highly coiled. A time consuming method of measuring transit through segments of the small intestine has been described by Kaus and coworkers (1986). They used a perspex capsule, containing technetium-99m labelled 'Amberlite' resin, and placed external markers on the front, back and sides of volunteers. The volunteers were imaged from the front, back and side which enabled the three dimensional movement of the capsule through the small intestine to be reconstructed and an estimate to be made of the velocity of the unit. After transit through the duodenum, which was too fast to be accurately measured, the capsule moved through the small intestine at between 4.2 and 5.6 cm per minute. There was no difference in transit times for two capsules with different specific gravities (1.0 and 1.6). The figure for rate of transit is in close agreement with the velocity of the migrating myoelectric potential down the small intestine (4.7 cm min^{-1}) measured by Kerlin and Phillips (1983) and that of 1 to 4 cm per minute for chyme (Granger *et al.*, 1985).

Read and coworkers (1986) have used a combination of scintigraphic, x-ray contrast and hydrogen breath techniques to follow the transit of a meal of sausages, baked beans and mashed potato. The residues left the small intestine between 2 and 12 hours after ingestion, suggesting that differential transit of meal components occurs; however, there is some controversy in the literature on this point. Kerlin and Phillips (1983) demonstrated a difference in transit between solids and liquids in the ileum whilst Malagelada and co-workers (1984) showed no difference in the small

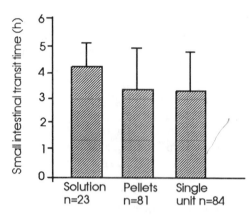

Figure 5.9.- Small intestinal transit times for
pharmaceutical dosage forms

intestinal transit time (S.I.T.T.) of the components of a mixed meal containing separately radiolabelled liquid and fibre. In the latter experiments, differences in mouth-to-caecum time of the two labelled components were entirely explained by differences in rates of gastric emptying. Caride (1984) determined a mean S.I.T.T. for a liquid test meal of 73 minutes, whereas our own comprehensive studies demonstrated a small intestinal transit around 4 hours for solutions, pellets and single unit formulations (Figure 5.9) (Davis *et al.*, 1986). Data from 201 studies have demonstrated that the S.I.T.T. of a dosage form is not affected by its physical state, size or the presence or absence of food, but high calorific loads may slow it slightly (Davis *et al.*, 1986).

A further intake of food appeared to have little effect on the transit of material already in the small intestine (Mundy *et al.*, 1989). Exercise also has been demonstrated to have no effect on small intestinal transit in normal subjects (Ollerenshaw *et al.*, 1987).

The studies to date show that the small intestinal transit time is remarkably resistant to pharmaceutical intervention and in man physical properties such as shape, density or putative bioadhesive properties are without significant effect on transit. Fats have been shown to have a minor effect on small intestinal transit though the effect on gastric emptying is considerably stronger.

RELATIONSHIP BETWEEN DRUG ABSORPTION AND POSITION OF DOSE FORM.
Radio Controlled Capsule
Zimmer and coworkers (1981) have described a capsule containing a balloon filled with drug which can be actuated at various positions in the gastrointestinal tract by application of a radio signal. This has been used to study absorption at various sites in the gastrointestinal tract. To locate the capsule, it is swallowed with a small dose of barium sulphate to aid its localisation within the gut and is triggered when required. In a study by Graul and coworkers (1985) the absorption of frusemide was compared in 5 subjects using the device. The drug was released in the ileo-caecal area in 3 subjects and in the ascending colon in the other two. Maximum plasma concentrations were lower after the release of the drug in the colon and there was a forty fold difference between absorption from the stomach and colon with bioavailabilities of 20% and 3% respectively. The capsule was also used to study the absorption of theophylline from the stomach, ileum and colon (Staib *et al.*,

1986). The mean relative bioavailability of theophylline was 86% after releasing the drug in the colon. Thus there was no evidence for a so-called absorption window for theopylline which has previously been reported in the literature, suggesting that such a "window" might have been related to the pharmaceutical formulations used. The device provides a means of investigating drug absorption under normal physiological conditions but has limitations of single occasion use and the need for repeated x-rays (Bieck, 1989).

Although in many studies there have been good correlations between the gamma scintigraphic data and the plasma concentration profile, there have been examples in the literature where the results have been completely inexplicable. Bogentoft and coworkers (1984) studied the absorption of acetylsalicylic acid from enteric-coated tablets in relation to gastric emptying and *in vivo* disintegration. Tablets were labelled with ^{51}Cr and transit followed in six healthy individuals in fasting and fed conditions by external scintigraphy. In eight of the 12 experiments, the time of onset of absorption correlated well with the time of disintegration. In four other experiments, three in postprandial state and one under fasting conditions, the absorption of acetylsalicylic acid was delayed more than 10 hours in spite of the fact that complete disintegration and gastric emptying of the tablet seemed to have occurred.

Absorption of Drugs and Foreign Substances through the Lymphatic System. The lymphatic route has been suggested as a method of by-passing first-pass metabolism for extremely lipid soluble drugs. It has been argued that lipophilic drugs may become incorporated into lipid micelles and transformed into chylomicrons by the epithelium before being released into the lymphatic circulation. All the lymph from the lower part of the body flows up through the thoracic duct and empties into the venous system of the left internal jugular vein, thus avoiding the hepatic portal system. In order to be transported in the chylomicrons, the drug must be extremely lipophilic. The ratio of portal blood flow to intestinal lymph flow in the rat is approximately 500:1. Although lymph is the major transport route for fats, it only contains 1% lipids. The overall effect is to make systemic absorption 50,000 times more efficient than lymphatic absorption. In order for a drug to be transported at equal rates by both lymphatic and systemic circulations, the drug must be 50,000 times more soluble in the chylomicrons than the plasma, i.e have a partition coefficient of 50,000 (log P = 4.7), which agrees with the suggested values of Noguchi and co-workers (1985).

As expected, in practice the lymphatic route is of little importance, except for those materials which are extremely lipophilic, for example insecticides such as dichlorodiphenyltrichloroethane (DDT), in which the loading of drug in the chylomicrons is as high as 0.6 to 2% by weight (Palin *et al.*, 1982; Vost and Maclean, 1984; Charman and Stella, 1986). These values are approximately 6 to 20% of the saturated solubility of DDT in triglycerides.

Studies of mesenteric lymph and blood plasma levels of *p*-aminosalicylic acid delivered intra-duodenally to rats suggested that drug was directly transported to the lymphatics (DeMarco and Levine, 1969). In addition, tetracycline was found in the central lacteal of the villi after administration, but this route was insignificant compared to the systemic absorption.

Gianninna and coworkers (1966) found that in the rat the absorption of oestradiol-3-cyclopentyl ether administered in an aqueous solution was mainly via the portal vein, but when the drug was given in sesame oil (primarily linoleic and oleic acid triglycerides) a greater proportion of the drug was absorbed by the lymphatic route. Addition of glyceryl mono-oleate to the sesame oil augmented this effect. The lymphatic absorption of probucol, a lipid-lowering agent, is also enhanced by food with high fat content, presumably to dissolve the drug in the fat prior to absorption (Palin *et al.*,1984). The natural extension of this is to dissolve the drug in a lipid administered as an emulsion, an approach which has proven useful with griseofulvin (Bates and Sequeira, 1975), although solubilization by bile salts may also be important for this material.

CONCLUSIONS

Transit through the small intestine appears to be remarkably constant at about 4 hours which is shorter than that quoted in most classical physiology texts. However, the length of stagnation of material at the ileocaecal junction is extremely variable. Although drugs are best absorbed from the duodenum, passage through this area is usually too rapid for significant drug absorption to occur. Several indirect methods have been employed to increase the contact time of a drug with the small intestinal surface, such as retention of the dosage form within the stomach which then trickles drug over the absorptive surface. This type of delivery, unfortunately, can only be successful when the subjects are fed, which can lead to complications of food-drug interactions.

REFERENCES

Bates T.R. and Sequeira J.A. (1975) Bioavailability of micronised griseofulvin from corn oil-in-water emulsion, aqueous suspension and commercial tablet dosage forms in humans. *J. Pharm. Sci.* **64** 793-797.

Bieck P.R. (1989) Drug absorption from the human colon. in "Drug Delivery and the Gastrointestinal tract" eds Wilson C.G., Hardy J.G. and Davis S.S. (Ellis-Horwood, Chichester). in press.

Bogentoft C., Alpsten M. and Ekenved G. (1984) Absorption of acetylsalicylic acid from enteric-coated tablets in relation to gastric emptying and *in-vivo* disintegration. *J. Pharm. Pharmacol.* **36** 350-351.

Borgström B. and Laurell C-B. (1953) Studies on lymph and lymph-protein during absorption of fat and saline in rats. *Acta Physiol. Scand.* **29** 264-280.

Bryan A.J., Kaur R., Robinson G., Thomas N.W. and Wilson C.G. (1980) Histological and physiological studies on the intestine of the rat exposed to solutions of Myrj 52 and PEG 2000. *Int. J. Pharmaceut.* **7** 145-156.

Caride C.J. (1984) Scintigraphic determination of small intestinal transit time: comparison with the hydrogen breath technique. *Gastroenterology* **86** 714-720.

Charman W.N.A. and Stella V. J. (1986) Effects of lipid class and lipid vehicle volume on the intestinal lymphatic transport of DDT. *Int. J. Pharmaceut.* **33** 165-172.

Davis S.S., Hardy J.G. and Fara J.W. (1986) Transit of pharmaceutical dosage forms through the small intestine. *Gut* **27** 886-892.

Davis S.S. (1989) Small intestine transit. in "Drug Delivery and the Gastrointestinal tract" eds Wilson C.G., Hardy J.G. and Davis S.S. (Ellis-Horwood, Chichester). in press.

DeMarco T.J. and Levine R.R. (1969) Role of lymphatics in the intestinal absorption and distribution of drugs. *J. Pharmacol. Exp. Therap.* **169** 142-151.

Gianninna T., Steinetz B.G. and Meli A. (1966) Pathway of absorption of orally administered ethynyl estradiol-3-cyclopentyl ether in the rat as influenced by vehicle of administration. *Proc. Soc. Exp. Biol. Med.* **121** 1175-1179.

Granger D.N., Barrowman J.A. and Kvietys P.R. (1985) The Small Intestine. in *Clinical Gastrointestinal Physiology* (Saunders, Philadelphia) **7** 141-207.

Graul E.H., Loew D. and Schuster O. (1985) Voraussetzung fur die Entwicklung einer sinnvollen Retard- und Diuretika-Komination. *Therapiewoche* **35** 4277-4291.

Hardy J.G., Evans D.F., Zaki I., Clark A.G., Tønnesen H.H. and Gamst O.N. (1987) Evaluation of an enteric-coated naproxen tablet using gamma scintigraphy and pH monitoring. *Int. J. Pharmaceut.* **37** 245-250.

Ho F.H.N., Merkle H.P. and Higuchi W.I. (1983) Quantitative, mechanistic and physiologically realistic approach to the biopharmaceutical design of oral drug delivery systems. *Drug Devel. Ind. Pharm.* **9** 1111-1184.

Kaus L.C., Fell J.T., Sharma H. and Taylor D.C. (1986) Representation of the path of a non-disintegrating capsule in the gastrointestinal tract using external scintigraphy and computer graphics. *Nucl. Med. Commun.* **7** 587-591.

Kellow J.E., Borody T.J., Phillips S.F., Tucker R.L. and Haddad A.C. (1986). Human interdigestive motility: variations in pattern from oesophagus to colon. *Gastroenterology* **91** 386-395.

Kerlin P. and Phillips S.F. (1983) Differential transit of liquids and solid residue through the human ileum. *Am.J. Physiol.* **245** G38-G43.

Kitizawa S., Ito H. and Sezak H. (1975) Transmucosal fluid movement and its effect on drug absorption. *Chem. Pharm. Bull.* **23** 1856-1865.

Lucas M. (1984) The surface pH of the intestinal mucosa and its significance in the permeability of organic anions. in *Pharmacology of Intestinal Permeation II.* : ed Csáky T.Z. Springer-Verlag, Berlin. pp119-163.

Malagelada J-R, Robertson J.S., Brown M.L., Remington M., Duenes J.A., Thomforde G.M. and Carryer P.W. (1984) Intestinal transit of solid and liquid components of a meal in health. *Gastroenterology* **87** 1255-1263.

Marvola M., Aito H., Pohto P., Kannikoski A., Nykanen S. and Kokkonen P. (1987) Gastrointestinal transit and concomitant absorption of verapamil from a single-unit sustained-release table. *Drug Dev. Ind. Pharm.* **13** 1593-1609.

Mundy M.J., Wilson C.G. and Hardy J.G. (1989) The effect of eating on transit through the small intestine. *Nucl. Med. Commun.* **10** 45-50.

Noguchi T., Charman W.N.A. and Stella V.J. (1985). The effect of lipophilicity and lipid vehicles on the lymphatic transport of various testosterone esters. *Int. J. Pharmaceut.* **24** 173-184.

Ochensfahrt H. and Winne D. (1974a) The contribution of solvent drag to the intestinal absorption of the acidic drugs benzoic acid and salicyclic acid from the jejunum of the rat. *Naunyn. Schmiedebergs Arch. Pharmacol.* **281** 175-196.

Ochensfahrt H. and Winne D. (1974b) The contribution of solvent drag to the intestinal absorption of the basic drugs amidopyrine and antipyrine from the jejunum of the rat. *Naunyn. Schmiedebergs Arch. Pharmacol.* **281** 197-217.

Ollerenshaw K.J., Norman S., Wilson C.G. and Hardy J.G. (1987) Exercise and small intestinal transit. *Nucl. Med. Commun.* **8** 105-110.

Pahlin P-E (1975) Extrinsic nervous control of the ileo-cecal sphincter in the cat. *Acta Physiol. Scand. Suppl.* **426** 1-32.

Palin K.J., Wilson C.G., Davis S.S. and Phillips A.J. (1982) The effects of oils on the lymphatic absorption of DDT. *J. Pharm. Pharmacol.* **34** 707-710.

Palin K.J. and Wilson C.G. (1984) The effect of different oils on the absorption of probucol in the rat. *J. Pharm. Pharmacol.* **36** 641-643.

Phillips S.F. (1983) Diarrhea: role of the ileocecal sphincter. In *New Trends in Pathophysiology and Therapy of the Large Bowel.* ed. Barbara L., Migioli M., and Phillips S.F. Elsevier Science Publishers BV, Amsterdam.

Phillips S.F. (1989) Transit across the ileocolonic junction. in *Drug Delivery and the Gastrointestinal tract.*eds Wilson C.G., Hardy J.G. and Davis S.S. (Ellis-Horwood, Chichester). in press.

Read N.W., Al-Janabi M.N., Holgate A.M., Barber D.C. and Edwards C.A. (1986). Simultaneous measurement of gastric emptying, small bowel residence and colonic filling of a solid meal by the use of a gamma camera. *Gut* **27** 300-308.

Simmonds W. J. (1954) The relationship between intestinal motility and the flow and rate of fat output in thoracic duct lymph in unaneasthetised rats. *Quart. J. Exp. Physiol.* **42** 205-221.

Staib A.H., Loew D., Harder S., Graul E.H., and Pfab R. (1986) Measurement of theophylline absorption from different regions of the gastro-intestinal tract using a remote controlled drug delivery device. *Eur. J. Clin. Pharmacol.* **30** 691-697.

Tasker R. R. (1951) The collection of intestinal lymph from normally active rats. *J. Physiol. (Lond)* **115** 292-295.

Taylor D.C. (1989) Models for intestinal permeability too drugs. in *Drug Delivery and the Gastrointestinal tract.* eds Wilson C.G., Hardy J.G. and Davis S.S. (Ellis-Horwood, Chichester). in press.

Toothaker R.D. and Welling P.G. (1980) The effect of food on drug bioavailability. *Ann. Rev. Pharmacol. Toxicol.* **20** 173-199.

Vost A. and Maclean N. (1984) Hydrocarbon transport in chylomicrons and high density lipoproteins in the rat. *Lipids* **19** 423-435.

Yoffey J.M. and Cortice F.C. (1970) in *Lymphatics, lymph and the lymphomyeloid complex.* Academic Press, New York and London.

Zimmer A., Roth W., Hugemann B., Spieth W., Koss F.W. (1981) A novel method to study drug absorption. Evaluation of the sites of absorption with a capsule for wire less controlled drug liberation in the gastrointestinal tract. *Technique et Documentation* Paris. pp. 211-214.

6

Drug Delivery to the Large Intestine

Karen P. Steed, Clive G. Wilson and Neena Washington.

The large intestine is responsible for the conservation of water and electrolytes, the formation of a solid stool and storage until a convenient time for defaecation. Unlike the small intestine, the residence time in the large bowel can be highly variable, ranging from as little as a few hours to as long as one week. In most individuals, dietary and social habits condition the time of defaecation. The majority of adults defaecate once a day, although frequencies from 2 per day to once every 2 days are considered normal.

Administration by the rectal route is preferable for drugs which produce emesis or are irritant when given orally. For the purposes of drug delivery, the colon has to be considered as two regions; the distal colon, which can be reached from the anus, and the proximal colon, which is only accessible via the oral route. The splenic flexure limits the area of exposure of drugs administered by the anal route to the descending and sigmoid colon, rectum and anus. Instillations of large volumes to overcome the restriction trigger the defaecation reflex. Nevertheless the rectal route is popular in Europe, though not in the U.S.A! Formulations targeted to the proximal colon have to be delivered via the oral route and must be protected against the hostile environment of the stomach and small intestine. Transit through the colon is slower than other areas of the gastrointestinal tract and therefore there is an opportunity for sustained drug delivery.

ANATOMY AND PHYSIOLOGY OF THE COLON.
The colon extends from the ileo-caecal junction to the anus and is approximately 125 cm long *in vivo*. It can be divided into the caecum, ascending, transverse,

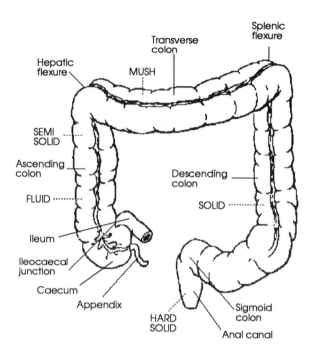

Figure 6.1. - Anatomy of the colon

descending and sigmoid colon, rectum and anus (Figure 6.1).

The caecum is the widest part of the colon and is a downward pointing blind pouch approximately 8.5 cm long with the appendix attached to its apex, and its base at the ileo-caecal junction. It is attached to the floor of the right iliac fossa by the peritoneum, within the folds of which lies the appendix.
The ascending colon is approximately 20 cm long and extends from the caecum to the hepatic flexure, which lies lateral to the right kidney and in contact with the inferior surface of the liver.
The transverse colon is normally over 45 cm in length and hangs loosely between the hepatic and the splenic flexures, often following the greater curvature of the stomach. The splenic flexure is usually located higher than the hepatic flexure.
The descending colon extends downwards from the splenic flexure to the pelvic brim and is approximately 30 cm long. The colon then turns towards the midline to form the coiled sigmoid colon, which is about 40 cm in length. This in turn joins the rectum in front of the third part of the sacrum and travels for approximately 12 cm before joining the anal canal. This is 3 cm long and is identified by the presence of the anal sphincters which replace the muscular coats of the rectum. The ano-rectal junction is supported by the sling of the *puborectales* muscle.

The wall of the colon is divided into four layers: serosa, *muscularis externa*, submucosa and mucosa. The squamous epithelium of the serosa is covered with fat distended pouches of peritoneum known as *appendices epiploicae*. These are larger and more numerous in the distal half of the colon and are one of its distinguishing features. The serosa is absent from the rectum and anal canal.

The *muscularis externa* consists of an inner circular muscle layer and an incomplete outer longitudinal layer composed of three separate 0.8 cm wide, longitudinal strips known as *teniae coli*. These bands converge in the caecum at the root of the appendix. They travel the length of the colon and eventually widen and join to form a continuous outer longitudinal muscle layer which covers the rectum. Between the *teniae coli* is a thin layer of longitudinal muscle which allows the inner circular muscle layer to bulge outwards. This outward bulge is interrupted at intervals by contractions of the circular muscle, giving the colon its characteristic sacculated appearance. These sacculae are known as haustra and are more pronounced in the proximal half of the colon. Their size and shape varies with the contractile activity of the circular muscle.

The submucosa of the colon contains many blood and lymph vessels, dense connective tissue which is sparsely infiltrated by cells such as fibroblasts, lymphocytes, plasma cells etc.

Colonic Mucosa

The colonic mucosa is divided into three layers: the *muscularis mucosae*, the *lamina propria* and the epithelium. The *muscularis mucosae* is a layer of smooth muscle approximately 10 cells thick which separates the submucosa from the *lamina propria*. The *lamina propria* supplies structural support for the epithelium and is well supplied with blood vessels and lymphatics. It also contains numerous T lymphocytes, macrophages, plasma cells and some lymph nodules. These cells play an important role in the immune function of the colon, and help to protect it from bacterial invasion and attack.

The epithelium consists of a single layer of columnar cells lining the colonic lumen, and is punctuated by numerous crypts. These are responsible for the production and differentiation of the absorptive, goblet and endocrine cells that make up this epithelial layer. The goblet cells are responsible for the production of mucus which is important in minimising friction between the mucosal surface and the semi-solid luminal contents.

Although there are no villi present in the large intestine, the mucosa is thrown into irregular folds known as *plicae semilunares* which, along with the microvilli of the absorptive epithelial cells, serve to increase the surface area of the colon by 10 to 15 times that of a simple cylinder of similar dimensions.

At the rectum there is a smooth transition in the outermost margins from smooth columnar epithelium to the stratified squamous epithelium of skin at the anal verge.

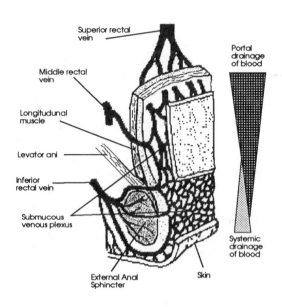

Figure 6.2.- Blood drainage territorries from the rectum

Blood Supply

The blood supply to the colon and upper rectum derives from the superior and inferior mesenteric arteries, and venous return is via the superior and inferior mesenteric veins (Figure 6.2). These join the splenic vein as part of the portal venous system to the liver. Thus any drugs absorbed from the colon and upper rectum are subjected to first pass elimination by the liver. Drugs absorbed from the lower rectum and anal canal are transported via the haemorrhoidal plexuses and internal iliac veins to the vena cava, and have the advantage of avoiding first pass elimination. This effect is reduced since the veins in this region are heavily anastomosed. In cases of portal hypertension, a significant proportion of a rectally administered drug can avoid first pass metabolism.

COLONIC ENVIRONMENT
pH

Work carried out by Evans and coworkers (1988) using a pH sensitive radiotelemetry capsule in normal, ambulatory volunteers has shown that the mean pH in the colonic lumen is 6.4 ± 0.6 in the right colon, 6.6 ± 0.8 in the mid colon and 7.0 ± 0.7 in the left colon. Disease or diet may alter the difference in pH between the right and left colon. Evidence exists suggesting that there are substantial changes in gastrointestinal pH in patients with malabsorption due to cystic fibrosis (Gilbert *et al.*, 1988). Current dosage forms designed for release in the proximal bowel employ enteric coatings, and are therefore dependent on luminal pH. Alteration of the pH profile of the gastrointestinal tract in various disease states may be an important factor influencing the bioavailability of drugs delivered in this form.

Bacteria

The colonic microflora contain up to 400 different species of both aerobic and anaerobic bacteria. The most prevalent anaerobes are *Bacteroides sp.* and *Bifidobacterium* whilst the most numerous aerobes are *Escherichia coli*, enterococci and *Lactobacillus*. The major site of bacterial activity is the caecum where the anaerobic bacteria ferment substrates in a liquid mixture. In man, the metabolic activity of the caecal bacteria can be demonstrated by ingestion of lactulose or baked beans which are fermented by the caecal bacteria causing a rise in breath hydrogen. This is used as a method of estimating the time of mouth to caecal transit.

Bacteria make up approximately 30% of faecal dry weight, and are responsible for the fermentation of dietary fibre and the carbohydrate components of mucus into short chain fatty acids (acetic, propionic and butyric acids), significant amounts of which are absorbed by passive diffusion and metabolised in the epithelial cells and liver (Cummings *et al.*, 1987). Short chain fatty acids remaining in the colon are neutralised by bicarbonate ions which are secreted into the lumen.

Colonic bacteria possess exocellular lipases which are able to hydrolyse fatty acid esters at the 1 and 3 positions of the triglyceride molecule. They also produce enzymes capable of metabolising long chain fatty acids. Approximately 25% of faecal fatty acids are hydroxylated by colonic bacteria, e.g. oleic acid is hydroxylated to form hydroxystearic acid. The presence of hydroxylated fatty acids in the colon has an inhibitory effect on colonic electrolyte and water transport, and at high concentrations they cause net secretion of water and electrolytes, which results in diarrhoea and therefore a significantly increased colonic transit rate. Spiller and coworkers (1986) showed that infusion of oleic acid (43 mg ml^{-1}) into the mid-ascending colon accelerated colonic transit rate and defaecation when compared to a control infusion.

Drugs such as stilboestrol, morphine and indomethacin are excreted in the bile as inactive sulphate or glucuronic acid conjugates. These conjugates are metabolised by bacterial enzymes to release the active form of the drug, which can then be reabsorbed and prolong pharmacological action (Peppercorn and Goldman, 1976).

Water and Electrolytes
The colon is responsible for the absorption of sodium ions, chloride ions and water from the lumen in exchange for bicarbonate and potassium ions. The absorption of sodium is an active process and involves its diffusion across the apical membrane of epithelial cells via water filled channels. A sodium-potassium exchange pump system in the baso-lateral membrane then moves sodium against steep concentration (14 mM to 140 mM) and electrical (-30 mV to +20 mV) gradients into the intercellular space. This movement of sodium creates an osmotic gradient which causes a net movement of water from the colonic lumen via the epithelial cells and through the tight junctions between epithelial cells into the intercellular spaces.

In healthy individuals, approximately 10 mEq of potassium enters the colon each day whilst 5 to 15 mEq are lost in the faeces during the same time period. Potassium secretion is determined by the luminal concentration of potassium, with concentrations of below 15 mEq leading to net secretion. This is accomplished by passive movement of potassium ions along an electrochemical gradient from plasma to lumen, and is facilitated by the tight junctions between epithelial cells which are highly permeable to potassium ions. The sodium-potassium pump in the basolateral membrane of epithelial cells creates a high intracellular potassium concentration (80 mM), of which only a small proportion is lost to the colonic lumen, since the apical epithelial membrane is essentially impermeable to potassium.

Mucus
Much of the colonic mucin is sulphated, the degree of sulphation being greater in the distal colon and decreasing proximally towards the terminal ileum (Filipe, 1979). Histochemical studies have shown a relative depletion of colonic sulphomucins in both ulcerative colitics and patients with Crohn's disease (Ehsanullah *et al.*, 1982). Desulphation of the mucus will alter the net charge on the mucin and therefore change physical properties rendering it more susceptible to bacterial sialase attack (Rhodes *et al.*, 1985).

COLONIC MOTILITY
Nervous and Humoral Control.
Parasympathetic supply to the colon is provided by the vagi to the proximal colon and pelvic nerves to the distal colon, whereas sympathetic supply is via the splanchnic and lumbar colonic nerves which supply the proximal and distal colon respectively. Axons from both branches of the autonomic nervous system impinge on the neurons of the myenteric plexus. Vagal stimulation initiates segmental contractions in the proximal colon, whereas pelvic nerve stimulation causes tonic propulsive contractions in the distal colon. Stimulation of either the splanchnic or lumbar sympathetic nerves causes the colonic muscles to relax.

Electrical Activity.
Changes in the electrical potential of the smooth muscle coat are often used to assess gastrointestinal motility. Two types of electrical activity have been recorded in the colon: i) slow wave activity and ii) spike potentials. The former consist of regular phasic depolarisations of the cell membrane which originate in the circular muscle layer of the transverse colon (Christensen *et al.*, 1969). When compared with that of the stomach and small intestine, colonic slow wave activity is of low frequency and irregular. The slow wave pacemaker in the proximal or transverse colon maintains regular and coordinated activity throughout the colon and appears, at least in the cat, to migrate towards the caecum (Christensen and Hauser, 1971; Christensen *et al.*, 1974). The retrograde propagation of slow waves in the proximal segment allows longer mucosal exposure for the intraluminal contents resulting in more complete absorption (Devroede and Soffie, 1973). In man, the dominant slow wave frequency is 11 cycles per minute in the transverse and descending colon, slightly less in the caecum, ascending and sigmoid colon, whilst that in the rectum is the highest observed in the gastrointestinal tract (17 cycles per min).

Spike potentials may be superimposed on the slow waves or may exist as bursts unrealted to slow wave activity. They are thought to initiate functional colonic contractions and spike bursts of long duration (<10s) increase after eating and may increase luminal transit. Short duration spike bursts (>3.5s) are seen in patients with constipation and are not associated with movement of the intestinal contents. Such contractions only occur when the membrane potential rises above a prevailing threshold level which is set by both neural and humoral mechanisms.

Patterns of Motility
There are two kinds of mechanical activity in the colon: propulsive contractions which are associated with the aboral movement of luminal contents, and segmental or mixing activity (Table 6.1). Segmental activity consists of local contractions which are usually effected by circular muscle and lead to the mixing of luminal contents, whereas propulsive activity is largely due to contraction of longitudinal muscle. In the colon, the predominant activity is segmental, with the propulsive type of movement occurring infrequently (3-4 times daily in normals).

Table 6.1. - Patterns of colonic motility (after Granger *et al.,* 1985).

	Frequency of occurrence			
Type of Movement	At Rest %	Postprandial %	Distance Travelled	Rate (cm/min)
Haustral shuttling	38	13	0	0
Haustral propulsion	36	57	5 - 10 cm	2.5
Haustral retropulsion	30	52	5 - 20 cm	2.5
Multihaustral propulsion	9	17	Variable	2.5 - 5
Peristalsis	6	8	18 - 20 cm	1 - 2
Mass	Rare	12	≥ 30 cm	5 - 35

There is also evidence that the menstrual cycle and pregnancy cause disturbances in gastrointestinal function. Transit is delayed in the luteal phase of the cycle, i.e. when serum progesterone levels are highest and thus progesterone may depress colonic motility (Davies *et al.,* 1986).

Transit
Whole bowel transit time is extremely variable, both within and between individuals, ranging from 0.4 to 5 days (Hinton *et al,* 1969; Kirwan and Smith, 1974). The greater part of both the transit time and the variability is, however, attributable to colonic transit.

Krevsky and coworkers (1986) used gamma scintigraphy to study the colonic transit of an 8 ml bolus of indium-111 diethylenetriaminepentaacetic acid (DTPA), delivered directly to the caecum via an orally passed tube. The marker emptied rapidly from the caecum and ascending colon with a mean half emptying time of around 90 minutes. Retrograde flow from the transverse colon to the ascending colon was rarely observed and this, together with prolonged stasis in the transverse colon and rapid ascending colon emptying, suggested that the transverse colon had a more important storage and faecal dehydration function than the ascending colon.

The data available concerning movement of material through the colon is largely confined to measurements of whole gut transit time, since few workers have followed the transit through the individual sections of the gastrointestinal tract in detail. A comparison of the residence times of a single unit in the ascending and transverse colon as measured by gamma scintigraphy at Nottingham is shown in Table 6.2.

Table 6.2. - Colonic transit of single unit dose forms

	Morning dosed	Morning dosed	Morning dosed	Evening dosed
	Fasted	Light Breakfast	Heavy Breakfast	
Ascending colon	3.6 ± 1.2	2.48 ± 1.45	4.8 ± 3.9	8.9 ± 4.34
Transverse colon	5.8 ± 2.9	-	-	11.25 ± 3.24

There is a large variability in the data, but in general, units administered prior to retiring for the night demonstrated a slower colonic transit than those dosed in the morning. A study by Metcalf and coworkers (1987) estimated that the average transit time from caecum to splenic flexure was 14 hours. A study by Parker and coworkers (1988) demonstrated that 50% of large units reached the splenic flexure within 7 hours of entering the colon and the size and density of such units had little effect on the transit times.

Hardy and coworkers (1985) have studied the colonic transit of a pressure-sensitive radiotelemetry capsule 25 mm long by 9 mm diameter, comparable to a size 000 capsule, and a radiolabelled multiparticulate system comprising of 0.5 to 1.8 mm resin pellets. Although both preparations entered the colon simultaneously, on average the capsule reached the transverse colon before 86% of the pellets (Figures 6.3 and 6.4). Colonic transit times for capsules varied from 17 to 72 h. The colonic muscular activity was shown to markedly increase postprandially; however, no resultant propulsion of contents was observed. The increased activity was attributed

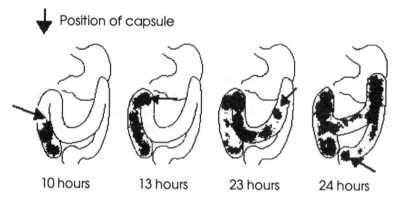

Figure 6.3. - Selective movement of a large unit ahead of small pellets in the colon

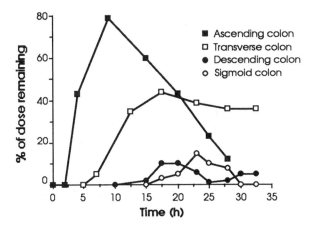

Figure 6.4. - Distribution of pellets within the colon

to the segmenting pattern of motility which caused the retention and mixing of small particles within the haustra whilst large indigestible particles passed through to the transverse colon. This selective retention of small particles is known as colonic sieving and is important in drug delivery, although the upper cut-off size limit for retention of particles have yet to be established. The sieving behaviour in disorders such as ulcerative colitis, where the degree of haustration is reduced, may influence the upper size limit for retention.

Gastrocolic Reflex
After eating, there is a rapid increase in colonic spike and contractile activity in the colon (Holdstock and Misiewicz, 1970; Wright *et al.*, 1980; Sun *et al.*, 1982) (Table 6.1). The calorific content appears to have a more important effect on the degree of motility than the size or pH of the meal. Fat is a more important stimulant than either carbohydrate or protein. Ingestion of fat alone produces both an early (10 to 40 min) and late (70 to 90 min) increase in colonic motility (Wright *et al.*, 1980). The late response was abolished by the simultaneous ingestion of protein, and both responses were inhibited by the ingestion of amino acids. This colonic response to feeding is known as the gastrocolic reflex, and must be an integrated response to both fat and protein induced mediators. The gastrocolonic response is initiated by a sensory receptor in the gastroduodenal mucosa (Sun *et al.*, 1982).

Tansy and Kendall (1973) distinguished three components in the response of the colon to the ingestion of a meal in dogs; an initial cholinergic propulsive reflex, followed by a cholinergic segmenting reflex and finally a noradrenergic segmenting reflex. Intravenous infusion of anticholinergic drugs prior to a meal abolishes the early colonic effects, thus supporting a cholinergic neural mechanism for mediation of the early response to eating. It is possible that there may also be a humoral component to this early response, in that the release of gastrointestinal hormones may be responsible for stimulating the cholinergic neural pathways. The late response, however, is unaffected by pretreatment with anticholinergic drugs, thus implicating an essentially humoral pathway which may involve release of gastrin, cholecystokinin (CCK) or another gastrointestinal hormone. A postprandial increase in gastrin levels has been observed and CCK is released from the duodenum in the presence of fat. Gastrin, in the G17 short chain form, and CCK stimulate colonic motility at serum concentrations within the normal range (Snape et al., 1978). Intravenous and intraduodenal amino acids stimulate the release of pancreatic glucagon, which has been shown to be a potent inhibitor of colonic myoelectric and motor activity. Enkephalins, endogenous pentapeptides, have been implicated since the response to a meal can be blocked by naloxone, an opiate antagonist (Sun et al., 1982). Met-enkephalin analogues inhibit colonic motility through a peripheral mechanism thought to involve the myenteric cholinergic plexus wheras leu-enkephalins stimulate motility through a centrally-acting mechanism (Vizi et al., 1984; Sun et al., 1982).

Recent studies at Nottingham (Bohemen et al., 1989) have shown that the increased colonic motility observed up to 4 hours postprandially is largely segmental. This implies that ingestion of food should not have any significant effect on the movement of drugs within the colon up to 4 hours after eating.

THE EFFECT OF DIET ON COLON PHYSIOLOGY.

The diet of an individual is closely linked with the proliferation of the colonic mucosa; food deprivation and "elemental diets' resulting in intestinal atrophy, and decreased cell production particularly in the colon (Janne et al., 1977; Goodlad and Wright, 1983). This is believed to be due to the lack of fermentable dietary fibre (Goodlad and Wright, 1983; Jacobs and Lupton, 1984). Goodlad and coworkers (1987) have shown that refeeding of starved rats with a fibre-free elemental diet supplemented with fermentable fibre stimulates colonic and small intestinal epithelial cell proliferation, whilst the addition of inert bulk to the elemental diet has no such effect. This proliferative effect of fermentable fibre on the gut epithelium was not observed in germ free rats, suggesting that epithelial proliferation is effected by the products of bacterial fermentation rather than the presence of fermentable fibre (Goodlad et al., 1989).

Colonic intraluminal pressure decreases after eating either wheatbran or cellulose (Findlay et al., 1974), however, physical characteristics of the dietary fibre may be important since coarse bran ingestion decreases colonic motility whereas ingestion of fine bran increases intracolonic pressure (Kirwan et al., 1974).

Diet, in particular dietary fibre, could therefore play a significant role in the absorption of drugs from the colon. Individuals ingesting a vegetarian diet or taking stool bulking agents may possibly show a difference in colonic drug absorption when compared with individuals ingesting a relatively low fibre diet. However, Cummings (1984) noted that increased dietary fibre led to decreased gastrointestinal transit times, which may offset any absorptive benefit gained by increasing the mucosal surface area in the colon. It is therefore expected that patients who have a predominantly vegetarian diet will show differences from the normal population with regard to the performance of sustained release formulations, predominantly due to differences in colonic transit. Scintigraphic studies have shown that in young vegetarians, mouth to anus transit of a single unit can be less than 6 hours; for one "normal" subject measured recently in our laboratory, the total transit time was 2 hours. A controlled release preparation for vegetarians thus represents a formidable challenge for formulators.

DRUG DELIVERY

After the hepatic flexure, the consolidation of faecal matter gradually increases the viscosity of the luminal contents with a resulting difficulty of diffusion of drug to the absorbing membrane. Therefore only in the ascending colon are conditions favourable for drug absorption.

Limited work has been carried out investigating the behaviour of pharmaceutical preparations in the colon, but present knowledge suggests that it is possible to optimise delivery systems for topical release of drugs to the colon, taking into account the predictable and nutritionally independent nature of small intestinal transit. The major problems are reduced surface area, wider lumen, sluggish movement, low volume of available dissolution fluid and the reduced permeability of the colonic epithelium to polar compounds. Thus it would be expected that the absorption of most drugs from the colon is slower than from the small intestine, but this is balanced by the longer residence time in this part of the gastrointestinal tract.

The importance of the colon as an area for drug absorption is illustrated in Figure 6.5 which shows the plasma concentration-time profiles of oxprenolol delivered in a Oros® device for two individuals with differing colonic transit times.

The Proximal Colon

Treatment of the proximal colon is problematic since penetration of a rectal enema is poor and only a small fraction passes the transverse colon even if the volume is increased to 200 ml (Hardy *et al.*, 1986). To achieve optimal colonic exposure, the drug has to be released as the formulation enters the caecum. If the drug is released prematurely, the majority would be absorbed from the small intestine and little would reach the colon. Eudragit and other enteric coatings are widely used to produce acid resistant formulations and with appropriate control of dissolution time may be reasonably effective in achieving release of drug in the ascending colon. More recently azopolymers have been examined as potential coatings which are degraded by colonic bacterial azo-reductase activity but are unaffected by acid conditions or the action of gastrointestinal enzymes (Saffran *et al.*,1986).

Once a drug has been released into the colonic lumen it is subject to possible metabolism by colonic bacteria, which may result in the release of toxic products or the metabolism of the active drug to an inactive metabolite. Studies by Magnusson and coworkers (1982) have shown that the bioavailability of digoxin from a delayed release formulation is reduced when compared with its bioavailability from conventional formulations due to its degradation by colonic bacteria to

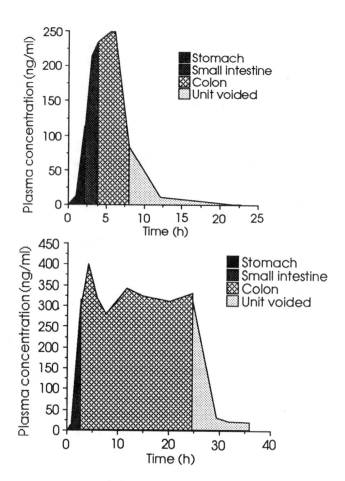

Figure 6.5. - Plasma levels of oxprenolol in two subjects with different colon transit times

the inactive dihydro-digoxin. However, some drugs, for example sulphasalazine, bisacodyl and the anthraquinones, used in the treatment of colonic disease, rely on the action of bacterial enzymes to release their active compounds. The diet of an individual can affect the colonic pH, since fermentation of carbohydrates may influence the metabolic activity of colonic bacteria and can lead to changes in drug bioavailability.

The sieving effect causes dispersible dosage forms such as pellets to become widely distributed in the colon whilst large single units or fragments of tablets travel rapidly through the colon ahead of the smaller pellets (Figure 6.3). This phenomenon is related to the observation that batches of markers of increasing sizes given with successive meals become interdispersed within the large intestine (Halls, 1965) which could be explained by the larger particles moving fastest. In the descending colon, the particles come together before defaecation. This data suggests that optimisation of drug delivery to the proximal colon may be achieved with a multiparticulate preparation which remains intact for approximately the first 5 hours after administration to the fasted patient. This would allow time for gastric emptying and transit through the small intestine. The drug preparation should then disperse allowing release of the material over the following 10 to 12 hours in the ascending and transverse colon. Extending the release profile over a longer period would not be an added advantage due to the variability of excretion patterns and the slower diffusion through consolidating faecal material.

Rectal Administration of Drugs
The rectal route is often used when administration of dosage forms by mouth is inappropriate, for example in the presence of nausea and vomiting, unconscious patients, if upper gastrointestinal disease is present which could affect the absorption of the drug, if an unpleasant tasting drug is used, and for gastro-labile drugs. In addition, the therapy can easily be discontinued and first-pass elimination of drug by the liver can be partly avoided. The absorption of drugs from the rectum has been contrasted with drug uptake from the duodenum (DeBoer *et al.*, 1984), however, since the rate of transit through the duodenum is extremely rapid, this is not a valid comparison.

Dosage Forms
Drugs can be administered in several formulations via the rectal route. Suppositories are normally either solid suspensions or solid emulsions, whereas rectally administered gelatin capsules can contain liquid formulations. Micro enemas have a volume of between 1 and 20 ml, and macro enemas 50 ml or more, both of which may be administered as either solutions or suspensions. The suspension suppository is the most widely used formulation, and it has been demonstrated that the release characteristics are dependent upon physiological factors, physicochemical properties of the drug, the suppository base and local environment within the rectum. In general, aqueous solutions of drugs are absorbed more quickly from the rectal route than the oral route, but absorption is usually slower with non-aqueous formulations, due to the limited amount of water available for drug dissolution.

Spreading of Dosage Forms.
In order to treat the colon via the rectal route, the preparation must spread efficiently. This limits topical treatment of the colon to areas distal to the splenic flexure. Retrograde spreading of foam enemas is less than for solution enemas, being limited to the sigmoid colon (Figure 6.6) (Wood *et al.*, 1985).

Tukker (1983) first described an elegant use of gamma scintigraphy to quantify the spreading of suppositories in recumbent dogs. The author constructed a series of activity profiles with time (Figure 6.7) to show the spread of Witepsol H15-containing suppositories with time. The results show that the addition of surfactants markedly affected *in vivo* spreading. Similarly preadministration of neostigmine which increases colonic motility markedly increased the spreading of the suppository.

Hardy and coworkers (1987) have described the spreading behaviour of suppository

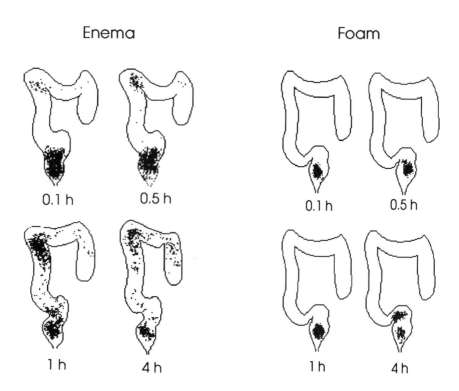

Figure 6.6. - Spreading of an enema and a foam after rectal administration

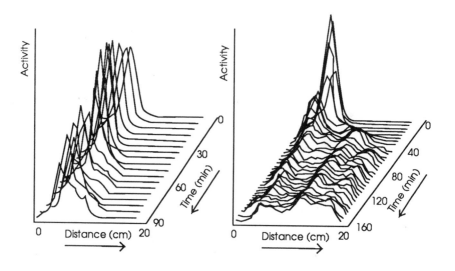

Figure 6.7. - Spreading of a Witepsol suppository activity-distance plots as a function of time, without (left) and with neostigmine (right) (after Tukker, 1983).

bases and incorporated suspension. The bases, Witepsol H15 and Labrafil WL2514, were labelled by the incorporation of small amounts of iodine-123 labelled unsaturated markers (arachis oil and Labrafil WL2700 respectively). The suspension consisted of micronised cationic exchange resin incorporated throughout the base at a disperse phase loading of 10% w/v. The results showed that most of the spreading of both base and suspension occurred in the first hour after administration and that the area of spreading was small with a maximum of 8 to 10 cm.

Therapeutic Agents
Formulations administered per rectum include foam and solution enemas and suppositories containing laxatives, soothing agents, corticosteroids such as hydrocortisone or prednisolone for treatment of inflammatory disorders. Anaesthetics and analgesics, e.g. thiopentone and methohexitone, are often rectally administered, since these compounds are very lipophilic and produce a rapid onset of action when administered by this route. Some benzodiazepines are also well absorbed rectally, e.g. diazepam, but etomidate does not produce adequate sedation when administered via this route. Rectal absorption of acetylsalicylic acid is strongly dependent upon the type of formulation in which it is administered, with an aqueous micro enema (20 ml at pH 4) giving the best results. In contrast, the pH of the paracetamol micro-enema is unimportant. Indomethacin and propionic acid derivatives are also well absorbed rectally. Narcotic analgesics are administered via this route when severe pain is associated with nausea and vomiting which makes oral administration impossible. However, the rectal route may not always be appropriate, for instance theophylline bioavailability is reduced when administered rectally.

Avoidance of First-Pass Metabolism
Venous return from the colon and upper rectum is via the portal vein to the liver. If a drug is delivered to the upper part of the rectum, it is transported into the portal system (Figure 6.2), and is therefore subject to first pass metabolism in the liver. The only way of avoiding first-pass metabolism is to deliver the drug to the lower part of the rectum. This simple principle is complicated by the presence of anastomoses which do not allow a precise definition of the areas which drain to the portal and systemic circulation. De Boer (1979) demonstrated a 100% increase in availability of lignocaine when administered rectally rather than orally, and it was calculated that the mean fraction of the rectally administered dose escaping first-pass metabolism was 57%. Other drugs with high first pass metabolism, such as salicylamide and propranolol, did not demonstrate a large increase in bioavailability when administered rectally; however, this may be due to incomplete absorption (De Boer, 1979; De Boer *et al.,* 1981), since these drugs exhibit a much larger bioavailability when administered rectally rather than orally to rats (De Boer, 1979; De Boer *et al.,* 1980, 1981).

Gut-wall metabolism of drugs is known to occur significantly in the upper gastrointestinal tract; however, its importance in the rectum is not known. Enzymes in the gut wall have a limited capacity, and their action can be saturated by large quantities of a drug thus effectively increasing drug bioavailability due to enzyme saturation.

Effect of Gastrointestinal Disease on Colonic Drug Absorption.
Gastrointestinal diseases are known to have a significant effect on the absorption of some orally administered drugs. Enteric coated formulations, designed for release in the colon, have been shown to release their contents in the stomach of achlorhydric patients. Such patients may have bacterial overgrowth in the small intestine which could lead to the premature release of drugs such as sulphasalazine or sennosides, thus rendering the therapy ineffective, as absorption would be complete before reaching the colon.

Patients with Crohn's disease are subject to gastrointestinal strictures where a controlled release matrix may lodge and cause epithelial damage due to the release of concentrated drug at one site over a prolonged period of time (Shaffer *et al.*, 1980).

Diarrhoea causes changes in the electrolyte content of the colonic lumen which therefore alters luminal pH, resulting in changes in the rate of absorption of drugs from the lumen. Diarrhoeal diseases cause decreased gut transit time and cause incomplete metabolism of pro-drugs such as sulphasalazine. The increased rate of transit would also be responsible for the premature voiding of sustained release formulations before complete drug release. It would also be expected to alter the sieving function of the colon.

CONCLUSIONS
Reliable delivery of drugs to the proximal colon is one of the key areas of research in drug delivery at the present time, which is hampered by the relative inaccessibility and the difficulty in producing in vitro models which mimic the environment of the colon. Results from the studies of sustained release dosage forms using pharmacokinetic and scintigraphic techniques indicate that for once a day dosing, the drug must be absorbed from the ascending colon to maintain therapeutic levels.

REFERENCES
Bohemen E.K., Steed K.P., Hardy J.G., Lamont G.M., Evans D.F., Wilson C.G. and Spiller R.C. (1989) Right sided colonic response to eating is largely non-propulsive. *Gut* **30** A749 - A750.

Christensen J., Caprilli R. and Lund G.F. (1969) Electrical slow waves in the circular muscle of cat colon. *Am. J. Physiol.* **217** 771-776.

Christensen J. and Hauser R.L. (1971) Longitudiinal axial coupling of slow waves in the proximal cat colon. *Am. J. Physiol.* **221** 246-250.

Christensen J. Anuras S. and Hauser R.L. (1974) Migrating spike bursts and electrical slow waves in the cat colon: effect of sectioning. *Gastroenterology* **66** 240-247.

Cummings J.H. (1984) Constipation, dietary fibre and the control of large bowel function. *Postgrad. Med J.* **60** 811-819.

Cummings J.G., Pomare E.W., Branch W.J., Naylor C.P.E. and Macfarlane G.T. (1987) Short chain fatty acids in human large intestine, portal, hepatic, and venous blood. *Gut* **28** 1221-1227.

Davies G.J., Growder M., Reid B. and Dickerson J.W.T. (1986) Bowel function measurements of individuals with different eating patterns. *Gut* **27** 164-169.

De Boer A.G. (1979) First-pass elimination of some high clearance drugs following rectal administration to humans and rats. PhD. Thesis, University of Leiden, The Netherlands.

De Boer A.G., Breimer D.D., Pronk J. and Gubbens-Stibbe J.M. (1980) Rectal bioavailability of lidocaine in rats: absence of significant first-pass elimination. *J. Pharm. Sci.* **69** 804-807.

De Boer A.G., De Leede L.G.J., Roozen C.P.J.M., Roos P.J. and Breimer D.D. (1981) Influence of the site of absorption in the rectum of rats on the bioavailability of high clearance drugs. *Federation Internationale Pharmaceutique Congress abstracts.* Vienna. p230.

De Boer A.G., De Leede L.G.J. and Breimer D.D. (1984) Drug Absorption by sublingual and rectal routes. *Br. J. Anaest.* **56** 69-82.

Devroede G. and Soffié M. (1973) Colonic absorption in idiopathic constipation. *Gastroenterology* **64** 552-561.

Ehsanullah M., Filipe M.I. and Gazzard B. (1982) Mucin secretion in inflammatory bowel disease; correlation with disease activity and dysplasia. *Gut* **23** 485-489.

Evans D.F., Pye G., Bramley R., Clark A.G., Dyson T.J. and Hardcastle J.D. (1988) Measurement of gastrointestinal pH profiles in normal, ambulant human subjects. *Gut* **29** 1035-1041.

Filipe M.I. (1979) Mucins in the gastrointestinal epithelium: a review. *Invest. Cell Pathol.* **2** 195-216.

Findlay J.M., Smith A.N., Mitchell W.D., Anderson A.J.D. and Eastwood M.A. (1974) Effects of unprocessed bran on colonic function in normal subjects and in diverticular disease. *Lancet* **i** 146-149.

Granger D.N., Barrowman J.A. and Kvietys P.R. (1985) Clinical Gastrointestinal Physiology. W.B. Saunders Company, Philadelphia.

Gilbert J., Kelleher J., Littlewood J.M. and Evans D.G. (1988) Ileal pH in cystic fibrosis. *Scand. J. Gastroenterol.* **23(Suppl. 43)** 132-134.

Goodlad R.A. and Wright N.A. (1983) The effects of the addition of cellulose or kaolin to an elemental diet on intestinal cell proliferation in the mouse. *Br. J. Nutr.* **50** 91-98.

Goodlad R.A., Lenton W., Ghatei M.A., Bloom S.R. and Wright N.A. (1987) Effects of an elemental diet, inert bulk and different types of dietary fibre on the response of the intestinal epithelium to refeeding in the rat and the relationship to plasma gastrin, enteroglucagon and PYY levels. *Gut* **28** 171-180.

Goodlad R.A., Ratcliffe B., Fordham J.P. and Wright N.A. (1989) Does dietary fibre stimulate intestinal epithelial cell proliferation in germ free rats? *Gut* **30** 820-825.

Halls J. (1965) Bowel shift during normal defaecation. *Proc. Royal Soc. Med.* **58** 859-860.

Hardy J.G., Wilson C.G. and Wood E. (1985) Drug delivery to the proximal colon. *J. Pharm. Pharmacol.* **37** 874-877.

Hardy J.G., Lee S.W., Clark A.G. and Reynolds J.R. (1986) Enema volume and spreading. *Int. J. Pharmaceut.* **32** 85-90.

Hardy J.G., Feely L.C., Wood E. and Davis S.S. (1987) The application of gamma-scintigraphy for the evaluation of the relative spreading of suppository bases on rectal hard gelatin capsules. *Int. J. Pharmaceut.* **38** 103-108.

Hinton J.M., Lennard-Jones J.E. and Young A.C. (1969) A new method for studying gut transit times using radio-opaque markers. *Gut* **10** 847-857.

Holdstock D.J. and Misiewicz J.J. (1970) Factors controlling colonic motility: Colonic pressures and transit after meals in patients with total colonic gastrectomy, pernicious anaemia and duodenal ulcer. *Gut* **11** 100-110.

Jacobs L.R. and Lupton J.R. (1984) Effects of dietary fibre on rat large bowel mucosal growth and cell proliferation. *Am. J. Physiol.* **246** 378-385.

Janne P., Carpenter Y. and Willems G. (1977) Colonic mucosal atrophy induced by a liquid elemental diet in rats. *Am. J. Dig. Dis.* **22** 808-812.

Kirwan W.O. and Smith A.N. (1974) Gastrointestinal transit estimated by an isotope capsule. *Scand. J. Gastroenterol.* **9** 763-766.

Kirwan W.O., Smith A.N., McConnell A A., Mitchell W.D., Falconer J.D. and Eastwood M.A. (1974) Action of different bran preparations on colonic function. *Br. Med. J.* **4** 187-189.

Krevsky B., Malmud L.S., D'Ercole F., Maurer A.H. and Fisher R.S. (1986) A physiological approach to the quantitative measurement of colonic transit in humans. *Gastroenterology* **91** 1102-1112.

Magnusson J.O., Bergdahl B., Bogentofot C. and Jonsson U.E. (1982) Metabolism of digoxin and absorptive site. *Br. J. Clin. Pharmacol.* **14** 284-285.

Metcalf A.M., Phillips S.F., Zinsmeister A.R., MacCarty R.L., Beart R.W. and Wolff B.G. (1987) Simplified assessment of segmental colonic transit. *Gastroenterology* **92** 40-47.

Parker G., Wilson C.G. and Hardy J.G. (1988) The effect of capsule size and density on the transit through the proximal colon. *J. Pharm. Pharmacol.* **40** 376-377.

Peppercorn M.A. and Goldman P. (1976) Drug bacteria interactions. *Rev. Drug Interact.* **2** 75-88.

Rhodes J.M., Gallimore R., Elias E. and Kennedy J.F. (1985) Faecal sulphatase in health and in inflammatory bowel disease. *Gut* **26** 466-469.

Saffran M., Kumar G.S., Savariar C., Burnham J.C., Williams F. and Neckers D.C. (1986) A new approach to the oral administration of insulin and other peptide drugs. *Science* **233** 1081-1084.

Shaffer J.L., Higham C. and Turnberg L.A. (1980) Hazards of slow release preparations in patients with bowel strictures. *Lancet.* **30 2 (8192)** 487.

Snape W.J. Jr., Matarazzo S.A. and Cohen S. (1978) Effect of eating and gastrointestinal hormones on human colonic myoelectrical and colon activity. *Gastroenterology* **75** 373-378.

Spiller R.C., Brown M.L. and Phillips S.F. (1986) Decreased fluid tolerance, accelerated transit and abnormal motility of the human colon induced by oleic acid. *Gastroenterology* **91** 100-107.

Sun E.A., Snape W.J., Cohen S. and Renny A. (1982) The role of opiate receptors and cholinergic neurones in the gastrocolic response. *Gastroenterology* **82** 689-693.

Tansy M.F. and Kendall F.M. (1973) Experimental and clinical aspects of gastrocolic reflexes. *Am. J. Dig. Dis.* **18** 521-531.

Tukker J. (1983) Biopharmaceutics of fatty suspension suppositories: The influence of physiological and physical parameters of spreading and bioavailability in dog and man: PhD thesis, University of Leiden, The Netherlands.

Vizi E S., Ono K., Adam-Zivi V., Duncalf D. and Földes F.F. (1984) Presynatic inhibitory effect of met enkephalin on [14C] acetylcholine release from the myenteric plexus and its interaction with muscarinic negative feedback inhibition. *J. Pharmacol. Exp. Ther.* **230** 493-499.

Wood E., Wilson C.G. and Hardy J.G. (1985) The spreading of foam and solution enemas. *Int. J. Pharmaceut.* **25** 191-197.

Wright R.A., Snape W.J., Battle W., Cohen S. and London R.L. (1980) Effect of dietary components on the gastrocolic response. *Am. J. Physiol.* **238** G228-232.

7

Drug Delivery to the Skin

Clive Washington* and Neena Washington
*Department of Pharmaceutical Sciences, Nottingham University,
University Park, Nottingham, NG7 2RD England.

The skin is the most extensive and readily accessible organ of the body. In an average adult, it covers a surface area of over 20,000 cm^2 and receives about one-third of the blood circulation. The skin is the common site of administration for dermatological drugs to achieve local action, and more recently it has also been used for the delivery of systemically acting drugs (Chien, 1983). A transdermal delivery device applies drugs in a small adhesive patch, which adheres to the skin and provides a sustained concentration of drug for absorption. Several drugs are administered by this route, notably scopolamine, glycerine trinitrate, clonidine and oestradiol.

STRUCTURE OF THE SKIN
The human skin consists of three anatomical layers (Figure 7.1):
i) the epidermis, which is a thin, dry and tough outer layer,
ii) the dermis, which is essentially the support system containing blood vessels, nerves, hair follicles, sebum and sweat glands,
iii) the subcutaneous fat layer which acts both as an insulator, a shock absorber and reserve depot of calories (Katz and Poulsen, 1971).

The epidermis is a multilayer consisting of two main parts: the stratum corneum and the stratum germinativum. The most superficial layer of the epidermis is the stratum corneum which consists of eight to sixteen layers of flattened, stratified and fully keratinised dead cells. Each cell is about 34 to 44 μm long, 25 to 36 μm wide and

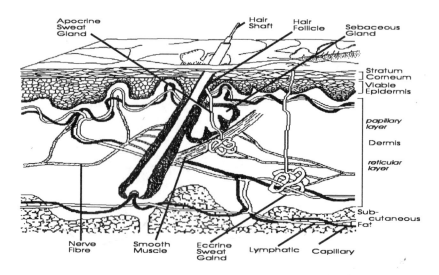

Figure 7.1. - Cross section through the human skin (redrawn from Katz and Poulsen, 1971)

0.15 to 0.20 μm thick. They are formed and continuously replaced by the basal layer of the stratum germinativum. The journey to the surface takes between 12 to 14 days, during which time the cells synthesise the various proteinaceous materials called keratin, and hence begin to die. The life span of such a cell on the surface is two to three weeks (Katz and Poulsen, 1971; Chien, 1982). The water content of the normal stratum corneum is 15 to 20% of its dry weight, but when it becomes hydrated it can contain up to 75% water.

The epidermis forms a barrier to water, electrolyte and nutrient loss from the body, and at the same time is also responsible for limiting the penetration of water and foreign substances from the environment into the body. Diseased, damaged or removed epidermis allows diffusion of small water-soluble, non-electrolytes to occur approximately 1000 times faster than in the intact skin (Scheuplein and Blank, 1971).

The dermis ranges from 2000 to 3000 μm thick and in man constitutes between 15 to 20% of total body weight. The dermis consists of a matrix of loose connective tissue composed of fibrous protein, embedded in an amorphous ground substance. There are two distinct layers in the dermis; the papillary layer, which is adjacent to the epidermis, contains mainly reticulin fibres, with smaller amounts of collagen and elastin. The reticular layer provides structural support, since it has extensive collagen and elastin networks, and few reticulin fibres.

The subcutaneous tissue of hypodermis is composed of loose, fibrous connective tissue which contains fat and elastic fibres. The base of the hair follicles are present in this layer, as are the secretory portion of the sweat glands, cutaneous nerves and blood and lymph networks (Figure 7.1). Most investigators consider that the drug has entered the systemic circulation if it reaches this layer; however the fat deposits may serve as a deep compartment for the drug.

The blood supply is located in the dermis. A deep plexus of arteries and veins is found in the subcutaneous tissue, and this sends out branches to the hair follicles and various glands. A second network of capillaries is located on the sub-papillary region of the dermis. From this plexus, small branches are sent towards the surface layers of the skin. The capillaries do not enter the epidermis, but they come within 150 and 200 µm from the outer surface of the skin. In man, blood flow is approximately 2.5 ml min^{-1} 100 g^{-1}, but it can reach 100 ml min^{-1} 100 g^{-1} in the fingers.

The hair shaft consists of differentiated, horny cells and it is the only part which breaks the surface of the skin. Hair follicles have a diameter of approximately 70 µm and occur at fixed intervals and hence this distance increases during growth. The density of hair varies over the body surface and it is absent from certain areas such as the lips and palms. The extent of hair growth plays an important role in fastening a transdermal system to the skin.

Sebaceous glands vary in size from between 200 to 2000 µm in diameter and are found in the upper third of the hair follicle. Sebaceous glands secrete sebum into the hair follicle, which eventually ends up on the surface of the skin. Sebum consists, on average, of 58% triglycerides, 26% waxy esters, 12% squalene, 3% cholesteryl esters and 1% cholesterol. The lipids maintain a pH of about 5 on the skin surface, and can cause problems for the adhesives in transdermal delivery systems.

Eccrine sweat glands are simple tubular glands which possess a coiled section located in the lower dermis. There are approximately 3,000,000 on the body. The normal diameter of the surface opening is 70 µm, but the average width of the ducts are between 5 and 14 µm. They make up 1/10,000 of the surface area. Eccrine sweat glands secrete fluid which consists of 99% water and other minor components. The pH of the secretion is about 5. Apocrine sweat glands are ten times larger than eccrine sweat glands and they open into the hair follicle. Apocrine glands secrete a lower volume of sweat than the eccrine glands, which consists of proteins, lipoproteins, lipids and several saccharides.

Nails are a modification of the epidermal structure. They are plates of hard keratin which lie along a nail bed, which is composed of modified skin and is very vascular.

The skin contains least moisture at its surface, 10 to 25%, with a pH of between 4.2 and 5.6. The lower epidermal layers contain up to 70% water and the pH gradually increases to 7.1 to 7.3. The "acid mantle" derives from the lactic acid and carboxylic amino acids in the sweat secretions mixed with the sebaceous secretions. The lower fatty acids (propionic, butyric, caproic or caprylic) have been demonstrated to have fungistatic and bacteriostatic action, possibly due to the low pH which they produce.

The isoelectric point of keratin is between 3.7 and 4.5 and hence materials applied to the skin should have a pH greater than this value.

PASSAGE OF DRUGS THROUGH THE SKIN

Topical application has been used for many centuries, mainly for the treatment of localised skin complaints. Usually, the drug only penetrates the outer layers of skin and little or no systemic absorption occurs. Transdermal delivery systems are specifically designed to enhance drug permeation into the systemic circulation.

Advantages and disadvantages.

The advantages of transdermal drug delivery have been summarised by Cleary (1984). Transdermally applied drugs avoid the chemically hostile gastrointestinal environment containing acid, food and enzymes. Consequently, this route is useful if there is gastrointestinal distress, such as vomiting. Since absorption of the drug does not take place in the intestine, the first pass effect is avoided. Patient compliance is good since a single application of the device can administer several days dose, and so is not subject to the problems of a schedule of tablet administration. Transdermal devices are usually well accepted, although they can cause irritation, the degree of which depends both on the drug and formulation. Finally, the devices have major pharmacokinetic benefits; they can provide a sustained plamsa profile over several days, without severe dips occurring at night, and without the potential for dose-dumping which can be a hazard with orally administered sustained release devices. Removal of the device causes the plasma levels to fall shortly thereafter, although some drugs can be stored in the hydrophobic regions of the skin and be released slowly into the blood.

There are several disadvantages, however; drugs may be metabolised by bacteria on the skin surface (Denyer *et al.*, 1985); epithelial bacteria can in fact be more prevalent under a transdermal device, since the increased hydration and uniform temperature can encourage growth. Enzymatic activity in the epithelium may be different to that in the gastrointestinal tract, leading to unpredictable routes of breakdown of drugs (Noonan and Wester, 1985). This may be useful since prodrugs can be administered which are metabolised to active species after adsorption (Bucks, 1984). The slow transport of many drugs across the skin limits this technique to potent drugs which require plasma concentrations of only a few micrograms per millilitre of plasma and which are not rapidly eliminated from the bloodstream.

These characteristics are ideally suited to for the delivery of peptides, which are digested in the gut and hence poorly absorbed orally. Peptides are not metabolised in the epidermis and are highly active in small quantities. However, they are normally too large and hydrophobic to be absorbed efficiently by this route. Some success has been achieved by using an electric field to drive peptides across the skin, a process termed iontophoresis. Chien and coworkers (1987) have had some success using this method for the transdermal delivery of insulin.

One of the primary functions of the skin is as a protective barrier to foreign agents and hence, it is not surprising that a complex relationship exists between the skin and the body's immune system. If an individual becomes sensitised to drug which has been delivered transdermally, it may become impossible to administer that drug by any other route (Lynch *et al.*, 1987). A number of cell types e.g. Langerhans cells and keratinocytes of the epidermis, indeterminant cells, tissue macrophages, mast cells, neutrophilic granulocytes and vascular endothelial cells of the dermis, are directly involved with the immune system. It is understandable that if the transdermal route of administration of a drug is chosen, there will be some stimulation of the immune system.

Maintaining contact between the device and the skin can present a problem. Application of the device occludes the skin, and this traps water and sebum from the glands. This, together with the flexing of the skin, can lead to loss of contact and discomfort. The choice of adhesive is restricted, since irritation must be minimised, and the drug must be transported through the adhesive. This was a problem during the development of many early devices, e.g. those for the delivery of clonidine. In many modern devices the adhesive is loaded with drug and becomes an integral part of the sustained release device. Finally, transdermal technology is often uneconomical compared to the simple oral tablet, and so is only used where specific advantages are gained.

Routes of absorption

Absorption can occur through several possible routes on an intact normal skin (Figure 7.2). It is widely accepted that the sebum and hydrophilic secretions offer negligible diffusional resistance to drug penetration. Drug molecules may penetrate not only through the skin but also via the eccrine glands and the sebaceous apparatus which is known as transappendageal absorption. This route is often neglected since it is difficult to study. The most useful technique is autoradiography of labelled drugs (Rogers, 1979). Since the openings of glands comprise only a fraction of a percent of the skin surface, transappendageal absorption is often considered unimportant; however it is likely that some materials do penetrate readily by this route. It has been suggested (Katz and Poulsen, 1971) that this route is more rapid than transepidermal transport, and so provides a loading dose, which is sustained by slower diffusion through the epidermis.

Drug diffusion from a transdermal delivery system to the blood can be considered as passage through a series of diffusional barriers. The drug has to pass first from the delivery system through the stratum corneum, the epidermis and the dermis, each of which has different barrier properties. Differences in composition of these layers cause them to display different permeabilities to drugs, depending on molecular properties such as diffusion coefficient, hydrophobicity, and solubility.

The first limiting factor is the vehicle or device in the case of transdermal systems. In a transdermal device, the primary design goal is the maintenance of the desired constant drug concentration at the skin surface for a suitable length of time. This has been achieved with a wide variety of technologies, and is the basis of controlled

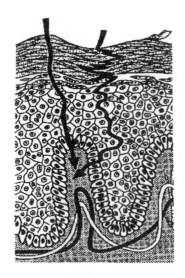

Figure 7.2. - Routes of penetration through the epidermis

transdermal drug delivery. This area has been extensively reviewed by Kydonieus and Berner (1987).

The second barrier consists of the stratum corneum. This dense, highly compressed layer is the principal barrier for most compounds. Monash and Blank (1958) showed that skin from which stratum corneum had been removed was highly permeable, while the removed stratum corneum was nearly as impermeable as the entire skin. Skin from cadavers showed approximately the same permeability as living skin, suggesting that the underlying tissues present little resistance to drug adsorption (Tregear, 1966). Transdermal drug absorption is influenced considerably by the degree of hydration of the skin. This is probably due to a combination of several factors including improved contact or wetting and hydration of the lipid channels of the stratum corneum. Even the application of oily materials can improve the skin hydration since evaporation of moisture from underlying tissues is reduced.

There are two possible routes of passage of drugs through the stratum corneum (Figure 7.2); these are the hydrophilic keratinised cells and the lipid channels between the cells. The lipoidal nature of the lipid channels favours passage of hydrophobic molecules and since many drugs are hydrophobic, this is their major route of entry. Behl and coworkers (1980) showed that hydration increased the penetration of polar molecules more than non-polar ones. Thus it is possible that hydration of the lipid channels is more important than hydration of keratinised cells.

The stratum corneum can act as a reservoir for drugs. This causes the pharmacological response to continue for a short time after the device has been removed. If the skin is then allowed to dry out, the drug will diffuse into underlying tissues more slowly, and application of an occlusive patch which rehydrates the skin can cause release of the drug at a later time.

The third barrier is the living portion of the epidermis and the dermis. Diffusion rates in these viable tissues are much higher than in the stratum corneum and consequently they offer little resistance to absorption. The tissues are much more hydrophilic than the stratum corneum, and so act as a barrier to hydrophobic compounds, which cannot partition into them.

MODELLING OF DRUG TRANSPORT ACROSS THE SKIN

A considerable amount of work has been performed on the mathematical modelling and quantitative understanding of the passage of drugs through the skin. Drugs pass by diffusion through three layers (the delivery device, the stratum corneum, and the epidermis) before reaching the blood. The model of Guy and Hadgraft (1985) is based on this three-layer structure and provides a quantitative description of drug absorption without a high level of complexity. The model is shown in Figure 3a. It is based around a number of simple assumptions; firstly that the drug passes by Fickian diffusion through the three layers, secondly that at each interface (device/ stratum corneum and stratum corneum/epithelium) the concentration ratio can be described by partitioning, and finally that the drug concentration in the blood is ef-fectively zero, i.e. the drug is removed rapidly when the end of the chain is reached. This model provides a good description of the behaviour of many simple drugs that do not undergo other processes (e.g. metabolism in skin, pro-drug transformation, etc.). Its predic-tions, without considering the detailed mathematics, can be illustrated by the diagrams in Figure 3 b,c and d.

Assume that the delivery system has been designed to maintain a constant concentration of drug at the device/skin interface, which will be the case in a well-designed transdermal device. A hydrophilic drug will only partition weakly into the stratum corneum and will not be transported easily across it. This is reflected in the sharp concentra-tion discontinuity at the device/skin interface and the rapid decay of concen-tration across the stratum corneum. However, at the stratum corneum/epi-dermis interface, the drug will partition into the hydrophilic epidermis and be transported easily across it. Note the small concentration discontinuity at this interface and the low slope of the con-centration profile in the epidermis. It is evident that in this case, stratum cor-neum transport is rate-limiting.

A hydrophobic drug (Figure 3c) will partition strongly into the stratum cor-neum at the interface with the device, and will be transported across the stra-

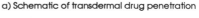

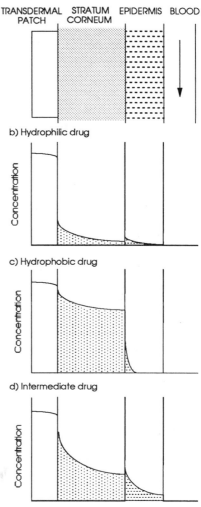

Figure 7.3. - Effects of hydrophobicity of a drug on penetration through the skin

tum corneum well. However, it will not partition into the epidermis due to its low solubility in this tissue, causing a large concentration discontinuity at this interface, and will not be transported efficiently through the epidermis.

Consequently, neither of these extremes are well absorbed transdermally, and it seems reasonable that a drug would be transported only if it can cross both hydrophilic and hydrophobic barriers, or have a 'balanced hydrophobic/hydro-philic character'. This situation is shown in Figure 3d. The drug is more hydrophilic than the extreme example considered in (b), so it partitions less well into the stratum corneum, and is transported more slowly across it. However, the drug reaching the stratum corneum/epidermal interface is sufficiently hydrophilic to partition into the epidermis and be transported to the blood.

This description is oversimplified and can be made more quantitative by specifying the rate constants for transport across the tissues and the partition coefficients. These rate constants can be measured *in vivo* and *in vitro*. Unfortunately, they are sensitive to intersubject variation in much the same way as other pharmacokinetic parameters.

PENETRATION ENHANCERS
A large number of materials have been applied to the skin in order to increase the penetration of other substances. These materials are known as penetration en-hancers. The use of differential scanning calorimetry (DSC) of the skin has contributed greatly to understanding of the mode of action of these substances (Barry, 1987). They are believed to operate by increasing the permeability of the stratum corneum, either in the lipid or the keratinised protein regions. It is unlikely that many materials penetrate to the epidermis in sufficient concentration to increase its ability to transport hydrophobic drugs.

Surfactants (Bettley and Donoghue, 1960) appear to assist the penetration of polar materials, and Bettley (1965) and Scheuplein and Ross (1970) proposed that their mode of action was on the keratinised protein regions of the stratum corneum. It is possible that a combination of hydration and protein conformational change is responsible for this effect. The most powerful surfactants, such as sodium dodecyl sulphate, denature and uncoil keratin proteins, leading to a more porous hydrated structure, through which drugs can diffuse more easily. However, strong surfac-tants may prove irritant if applied to the skin for long periods,

The largest class of penetration enhancers appear to fluidise the lipid channels. These include dimethyl sulphoxide (DMSO) at high concentrations, decylmethyl sulphoxide, and Azone. These materials are known to influence lipid structure (Beastall *et al.*, 1988) but are also polar and capable of swelling proteinaceous regions. This provides an indication of the importance of lipid fluidity, since at low concentrations substances such as DMSO swell keratin but do not appreciably improve absorption. Only at high surface concentrations (>60%) does DMSO affect skin lipid fluidity, accompanied by an increase in drug penetration.

Certain penetration enhancers, such as propylene glycol, assist other enhancers to enter the skin. For example, Azone is more soluble in propylene glycol than water, so propylene glycol assists its penetration. Additionally, propylene glycol may hydrate keratinised regions of the stratum corneum. Consequently, the Azone/ propylene glycol mixture is one of the most efficient of currently used penetration enhancers.

A fundamental difficulty with the development of penetration enhancers is that an attempt is being made to alter the skin structure; this is almost certain to provoke an irritant reaction. Both sodium dodecyl sulphate and DMSO are irritant; Azone is probably the least irritant, partly since it is active at low (1%) concentrations. This problem is made more severe since minor irritation is often found in transdermal therapy even before penetration enhancers are used.

FACTORS AFFECTING PERCUTANEOUS ABSORPTION.
Individual variation
Individual variation can be as severe a problem as for other drug delivery systems. Maibach (1976) studied the absorption of hydrocortisone in 18 males and found a range of absorption values varying nearly by ten-fold. Thus dosage must be titrated to achieve a therapeutic benefit and the transdermal system does have the advantage in this respect that treatment can be stopped rapidly if too great a response is observed.

Age
Skin condition and structure varies with age. The stratum corneum is not fully developed in neonates and this has been used to advantage in the administration of transdermal theophylline. It can also pose a major problem since externally applied materials, such as antiseptics and disinfectants, can be absorbed easily. Pre-term infants have very little barrier function, which does not develop until 9 months after conception. In older patients the stratum corneum thickens and is less hydrated, increasing its barrier function.

Site
Drug absorption varies greatly with site of application (Wester and Maibach, 1987). Thus hydrocortisone was found to penetrate the scrotum 40 times more rapidly than the forearm or back, which are commonly used application sites. Heavily keratini- sed sites, notably the arch of the foot, are several times less efficient than the forearm. This pattern appears to apply to most drugs and offers the interesting possibility of titrating the dose by varying the position of the transdermal device. However, it also poses problems since some patients experience minor irritation which encourages them to move the device.

Occlusion
Occlusion increases adsorption considerably in may cases (Feldmann and Maibach, 1965). This is probably due to increased hydration of the stratum corneum, leading to improved permeability to both polar and non-polar drugs.

Temperature

Temperature affects drug penetration by two mechanisms. Firstly it alters the physiology of the skin, and secondly the physicochemical diffusion rates increase with temperature. The skin temperature is strongly influenced by its surroundings, and may be 20°C cooler than body temperature or several degrees hotter. This is also linked to diseased states in which the body temperature may vary. Roberts and coworkers (1978) have found that temperature-induced variations in the diffusion coefficient may alter the absorption rate by up to a factor of two over this temperature range. Fortunately many transdermal patches act as insulators and so the observed range is likely to be lower in practice. The external temperature is more likely to influence the diffusion rate in the controlled release system itself.

Temperature also influences blood flow in the surface vasculature and so might be expected to influence adsorption through this route. However, this possibility has not yet been proven (Arita *et al.*, 1970).

Race

Race appears to influence penetration to a small extent. Negroid stratum corneum has more layers and is generally less permeable, although there is no difference in thickness between negroid and European stratum corneum (Weingand *et al.*, 1980). It is not known if the presence of melanocytes influences penetration of drugs.

Disease

The skin is the part of the body which comes into direct contact with the environment and hence it is usually the first part of the body to sustain damage or be exposed to irritant substances. Dermatitis is thus a fairly common complaint. The symptoms generally begin as itching, sweat production, increased sensitivity and pain, but lead to swelling, oozing, crusting and scaling, with thickening and hyperpigmentation. Inflammation occurs in response to a number of factors, e.g. mechanical, chemical, thermal stimuli, infections or imbalance in the autoregulation processes. All these processes can reduce barrier action and lead to increased permeability of the skin to drugs.

Skin permeability is increased in psoriasis (Carr and Tarnowski, 1968) and ichthyosis (Frost *et al.*, 1968). This is unusual since both of these conditions result in thickening of the stratum corneum; presumably it does not retain structural integrity.

Irritation and inflammation increase penetration even if the skin layer is unbroken (Spruit, 1970); ultraviolet light and sunburn also increase permeability. Burning from more conventional sources such as scalding causes greater penetration, the extent increasing with burn temperature but not apparently with burn duration (Behl *et al.*, 1980).

CONCLUSIONS.

Transdermal delivery has a number of advantages which can be of considerable value, most notably the ability to provide uniform plasma levels for considerable periods of time and avoidance of first-pass elimination. It also has disadvantages which are common to other delivery routes, such as intersubject variability and susceptibility to diseased states at the absorption site. At present, however, its main disadvantage is that only low plasma levels of drug can be maintained, and so it is limited to highly active drugs.

Despite these problems it is currently the optimal route for several compounds, and a number of commercial devices are well-established. It appears that transdermal delivery will be a valuable option in the development of future drug delivery systems.

REFERENCES

Arita T., Hori R., Anmo T., Washitake M., Akatsu M. and Yajima T. (1970) Studies on percutaneous absorption of drugs. *Chem. Pharm. Bull.* **18** 1045-1049.

Barry B.W. (1987) Mode of action of penetration enhancers in human skin. *J. Controlled Release* **6** 85-97.

Beastall J.C., Washington C. and Hadgraft J. (1988) The effect of Azone on lipid bilayer fluidity and transition temperature. *Int. J. Pharmaceut.* **48** 207-213.

Behl C.R., Flynn G.L., Kurihara T., Smith W., Giatmaitan O., Higuchi W.I., Ho N.F.H. and Peirson C.L. (1980) Permeability of thermally damaged skin. I. Immediate influences of 60°C scalding on hairless mouse skin. *J. Invest. Dermatol.* **75** 340-345.

Behl C.R., Flynn G.L., Kurihara T., Harper N., Smith W., Higuchi W.I., Ho N.F.H. and Pierson C.L. (1980) Hydration and percutaneous absorption 1. Influence of hydration on alkanol permeation through hairless mouse skin. *J. Invest. Dermatol.* **75** 346-352.

Bettley F.R. (1965) The influence of detergents and surfactants on epidermal permeability. *Br. J. Dermatol.* **77** 98-100.

Bettley F.R. and Donohue E. (1960) Effect of soap on the diffusion of water through the isolated human epidermis. *Nature (London)* **185** 17-20.

Bucks D.A.W. (1984) Skin structure and metabolism: relevance to the design of cutaneous therapeutics. *Pharm. Res.* **1** 148-153.

Carr R.D. and Tarnowski W.M. (1968) Percutaneous absorption of corticosteroids. *Acta Dermato-venerol.* **48** 417-428.

Chien Y.W. (1982) *Novel drug delivery systems.* Marcel Dekker, New York.

Chien Y.W. (1983) Logics of transdermal controlled drug administration. *Drug. Dev. Ind. Pharm.* **9** 9-34.

Chien Y.W., Siddiqui O., Sun Y., Shi W.M. and Lui J.C. (1987) Transdermal iontophoretic delivery of therapeutic peptides/proteins. *Ann. New York Acad. Sci.* **507** 32-51.

Cleary G.W. (1984) Transdermal Controlled Release Systems. In: Langer R.S. and Wise D.L. (eds), *Medical Applications of Controlled Release*, Volume I. CRC Press Boca Raton, Florida, pp 203-251.

Denyer S.P., Guy R.H., Hadgraft J. and Hugo W.B. (1985) The microbial degradation of topically applied drugs. *Int. J. Pharmaceut.* **26** 89-97.

Feldmann R.J. and Maibach H.I. (1965) Penetration of ^{14}C cortisone through normal skin. *Arch. Dermatol.* **91** 661-666.

Frost P., Weinstein G.D., Bothwell J. and Wildnauer R. (1968) Ichthyosiform dermatoses. III. Studies of transepidermal water loss. *Arch. Dermatol.* **98** 230-233.

Guy R.H. and Hadgraft J. (1985) The prediction of plasma levels of drugs following transdermal application. *J. Controlled Release* **1** 177-182.

Katz M. and Poulsen B.J. (1971) Absorption of drugs through the skin. in: Brodie B.B. and Gilette J.R. (eds), *Handbook of experimental pharmacology*, New Series, 28 Part 1, Springer-Verlag, Berlin. 103-174.

Kydonieus A.F. and Berner B. (1987) *Transdermal delivery of drugs.* (3 vols.) CRC Press, Boca Raton, Florida.

Lynch D.H., Roberts L.K. and Daynes R.A. (1987) Skin immunology: the Achilles heel to transdermal drug delivery. *J. Controlled Release* **6** 39-50.

Maibach H.I. (1976) In vivo percutaneous penetration of corticoids in man and unresolved problems in their efficacy. *Dermatologica* Suppl. **152** 11-25.

Monash S. and Blank H. (1958) Location and reformation of the epithelial barrier to water vapour. *A.M.A. Arch. Dermatol.* **78** 710-714.

Noonan P.K and Wester R.C. (1985) Cutaneous metabolism of xenobiotics. in: *Percutaneous absorption.* ed. Bronaugh R.L. and Maibach H.I. Marcel Dekker, New York, 65-85.

Roberts M.S., Anderson R.A., Swarbrick J. and Moore D.E. (1978) The percutaneous absorption of phenolic compounds: the mechanism of diffusion across the stratum corneum. *J. Pharm. Pharmacol.* **30** 486-490.

Rogers A.W. (1979) *Techniques of autoradiography.* Elsevier, Amsterdam.

Scheuplein R.J. and Blank I.H. (1971) Permeability of the skin. *Physiol. Rev.* **51** 702-747.

Scheuplein R.J. and Ross L. (1970) Effect of surfactants and solvent on the permeability of epidermis. *J. Soc. Cosmet. Chem.* **21** 853-857.

Spruit D. (1970) Evaluation of skin function by the alkali application technique. *Curr. Probl. Dermatol.* **3** 148-153.

Tregear R.T. (1966) *Physical function of skin* Vol 1. Academic Press, London.

Weingand D.A., Haygood C., Gaylor J.R. and Anglin J.H. (1980) Racial variations in the cutaneous barrier. in: *Current concepts in cutaneous toxicity.* ed. Drill V.A. and Lazar P. Academic Press, New York, pp221-235.

Wester R.C. and Maibach H.I. (1987) Clinical considerations for transdermal therapy. in: *Transdermal delivery of drugs.* eds. Kydonieus A.F. and Berner B. Vol 1 chapter 6, CRC Press, Boca Raton, Florida, pp71-78.

8

Ocular Drug Delivery

Jane L. Greaves

The external eye is readily accessible for drug administration; however, as a consequence of its function as the visual apparatus, mechanisms are strongly developed for the clearance of foreign materials from the cornea to preserve visual acuity. This presents problems in the development of formulations for ophthalmic therapy.

Systemic administration of a drug to treat ocular disease would require a high concentration of circulating drug in the plasma to achieve therapeutic quantities in the aqueous humour, with the increased risk of side effects. Topical administration is more direct, but conventional preparations of ophthalmic drugs, such as ointments, suspensions, or solutions, are relatively inefficient as therapeutic systems. A large proportion of the topically applied drug is immediately diluted in the tear film and excess fluid spills over the lid margin and the remainder is rapidly drained into the nasolacrimal duct. A proportion of the drug is not available for therapeutic action since it binds to the surrounding extraorbital tissues. In view of these losses frequent topical administration is necessary to maintain adequate drug levels.

Three factors have to be considered when drug delivery to the eye is attempted. Firstly, how to cross the blood-eye barrier (systemic to ocular) or cornea (external to ocular) to reach the site of action; secondly, how to localize the pharmacodynamic action at the eye and minimise drug action on other tissues, and finally, how to prolong the duration of drug action such that the frequency of drug administration can be reduced.

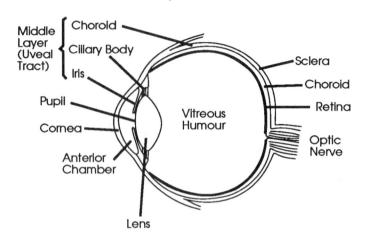

Figure 8.1. - Vertical section through the human eye

STRUCTURE OF THE EYE

The outer shape of the eye comprises of two spheres of different radii, one set into the other (Figure 8.1). The anterior sphere, the cornea, is the smaller and more curved of the two and is completely transparent. The posterior sphere or sclera is a white, opaque, fibrous shell which encloses the ocular structures. Both tissues are relatively nondistensible and protect the eye from physical damage.

The outer tissues of the eye consist of three layers: the outermost layer, the sclera and cornea, provide protection for the delicate structures within. The middle layer, the uveal tract, has a nutritive function, being mainly vascular and consisting of the choroid, ciliary body and the iris. The innermost layer is the retina containing photoreceptors and is concerned with the reception of visual stimuli. The inner eye is divided by the lens which separates the aqueous and vitreous humours. The iris separates the aqueous humour into the anterior and posterior chambers.

The Cornea

Even though the cornea covers only one-sixth of the total surface area of the eyeball it is considered to be the main pathway for the permeation of drugs into the intraocular tissues. The mean thickness of the cornea in man is just over 0.5 mm in the central region, becoming 50% thicker towards the periphery.

The cornea is made up of the stroma (up to 90% of its thickness) which is bounded externally by epithelium and the Bowman's membrane, and internally by Descemet's membrane and the endothelium (Figure 8.2). The corneal epithelium is composed of five to six layers of cells, increasing to eight to ten at the periphery with a total thickness of 50 - 100 μm. The cells at the base are columnar, but as they are squeezed forward by new cells, they become flatter so that three groups of cells are usually identified: basal cells, an intermediate zone of 2 - 3 layers of polygonal cells (wing shaped) and squamous cells. The permeability of the intact corneal epithelium is low until the outermost layer is damaged, suggesting that tight junctions exist between the cells of the outer layer. The outer layer of the surface cells possess microvilli on their anterior surface which presumably help to anchor the precorneal tear film. The cells of the basal layer show extensive lateral interdigitation of plasma membranes and are therefore relatively permeable (Pedler, 1962).

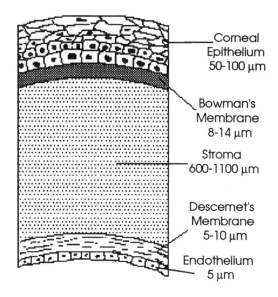

Corneal
Epithelium
50-100 μm

Bowman's
Membrane
8-14 μm

Stroma
600-1100 μm

Descemet's
Membrane
5-10 μm

Endothelium
5 μm

Figure 8.2. - The five layers of the cornea

Immediately adjacent to the epithelium is a less ordered region of the stroma, 8 - 14 μm thick, the Bowman's membrane. The layer is not sharply differentiated from the remainder of the stroma beneath it and could be described as Bowman's layer rather than Bowman's membrane (Kayes and Holmberg, 1960).

The stroma or *substantia propria* consists of collagenous lamellae running parallel with the surface and superimposed on each other. The lamellae are made up of fibres which run parallel to form sheets. The stroma can be considered to have a comparatively open structure which normally allows diffusion of solutes having molecular weight below 500,000 Daltons. It can act as a barrier for very lipophilic substances which pass freely through the epithelium, while it is easily penetrated by hydrophilic solutes.

On the interior surface of the stroma there is a 5 to 10 μm thick layer, Descemet's membrane, which is secreted by the endothelium. The endothelium consists of a single layer of flattened cells 5 μm high and 20 μm wide. These cells form a regular mosaic, with close contact between them. The endothelium is about 200 times more permeable than the epithelium and thus represents a weak barrier. The endothelium is in contact with the aqueous humour of the anterior chamber. The endothelial layer is crossed by a passive flux of water towards the stroma, which has a tendency to swell. An active pump mechanism generates a flux in the opposite direction which controls corneal turgescence (Maurice, 1972).

The Conjunctiva and Sclera

The conjunctiva line the posterior surface of the eyelids and cover the exterior surface of the cornea. The conjunctiva lining the lids is vascular (*palpebral conjunctiva*) and that on the globe is transparent (*bulbar conjunctiva*). The area between the lids and the globe is termed the conjunctival sac which is open at the front at the palpebral fissure and only complete when the eyes are closed.

The sclera forms the posterior five sixths of the protective coat of the eye. It's anterior portion is visible and constitutes the white of the eye. Attached to the sclera are the extraocular muscles. Through the sclera pass the nerves and the blood vessels that penetrate into the interior of the eye. At its most posterior portion, the site of attachment of the optic nerve, the sclera becomes a thin sieve like structure, the *lamina cribrosa*, through which the retinal fibres leave the eye to form the optic nerve. The episcleral tissue is a loose connective and elastic tissue that covers the sclera and unites it with the conjunctiva above.

The Eyelids

The eyelids are movable folds of modified skin consisting of orbital and palpebral portions positioned in front of the eyeball (Figure 8.3). They have an obvious protective function and also play an important role in the maintenance of the tear film and lacrimal drainage. Fibrous tarsal plates provide the framework for the lids.

The palpebral parts of the *obicularis oculi* muscle, particularly of the upper lid, are used in gentle lid closure, and the orbital parts are also brought into play in forcible lid closure. Closure of the lids is associated reflexly with an upwards movement of the eye which is effective before the lids are fully closed (Bell's phenomenon). The *orbicularis* muscle aids tear drainage and deep to this muscle is the tissue plane that contains the vascular and nervous supply to the lids. Closure of the upper lid by the *orbicularis* muscle is opposed by the combined actions of the striated *levator palpebrae superioris* muscle and its associated superior palpebral muscle which retracts the lid.

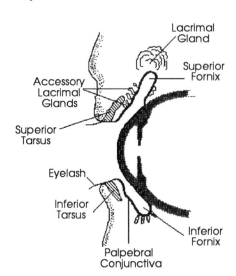

Figure 8.3. - Vertical section through the eyelids and conjunctiva

The Precorneal Tear Film

The precorneal tear film is a very thin fluid layer continuously bathing the corneal epithelium, the conjunctiva and walls of the conjunctival cul-de-sac. Normal secretion of tears by the lacrimal system is necessary for nutrition of the cornea, protection against bacterial infec-

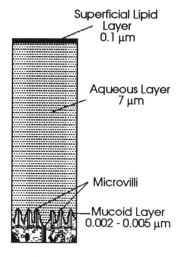

Figure 8.4. - The structure of the precorneal tear film

tion, the removal of cellular debris and foreign matter, and for the formation of a stable, continuous fluid film over the cornea producing a high quality optical surface.

The maintenance of a clear, healthy cornea requires that the anterior surface of its epithelial layer be kept moist. The moisture also provides lubrication for the movement of the eyelids. As the tear layer is so thin, evaporation and lipid contamination of the tear fluids' mucin component quickly destroys its continuity. This results in dry spots that appear usually within 15 to 30 seconds after a blink, at scattered locations on the corneal surface. The blinking action of the eyelids, which usually occurs before the actual formation of dry spots, is required to re-form the tear film layer. The blink interval should therefore, be shorter than the tear break-up time.

Wolff (1946) first described the precorneal tear film as a three layered structure. These layers are: the superficial oily layer, the middle aqueous layer, and the adsorbed mucus layer (Figures 8.4) which are secreted by several glands (Figure 8.5).

(i) *The Superficial Oily Layer* is approximately 0.1 μm thick and consists of wax and cholesterol esters secreted by the Meibomian glands, the glands of Zeis at the palpebral margin of each eyelid, and the glands of Moll situated at the root of each lash. This layer reduces the evaporation from the underlying aqueous phase by 10

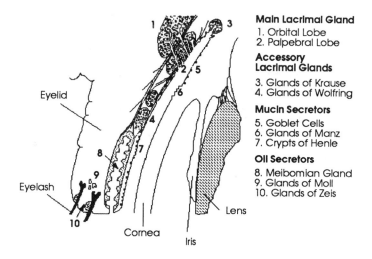

Figure 8.5. - The glands secreting the components of the precorneal tear film

to 20 fold, preventing the cornea from drying out (Mishima and Maurice, 1961; Mishima, 1965).

(ii) *The Aqueous Layer* lies below the oily layer and is the largest component of the tear film (6-10 μm thick), consisting of watery lacrimal secretions provided by the numerous accessory lacrimal glands of Kraus and Wolfring, most of which are situated in the upper conjunctival fornix.

(iii) *The Mucoid Layer* is secreted by conjunctival goblet cells, the crypts of Henlé which are situated on the conjunctival surface of the upper and lower tarsus, and the glands of Manz positioned in a circular ring on the limbal conjunctiva. Mucin is involved in adhesion of the aqueous phase to the underlying cornea, and thus keeps the cornea wettable.

The average human tear volume is 7 μl, 1 μl of which is contained in the precorneal tear film, and 3 μl in each of the tear margins (Shell, 1982). Prior to blinking, the tear volume can increase to about 30 μl. The maximum amount of fluid that can be held in the conjunctival sac is only about 10 μl. When the tear volume is suddenly increased, following the instillation of an eyedrop, rapid reflex blinking quickly re-establishes the normal tear pool. Most of the eyedrop is pumped through the lacrimal drainage system into the nasolacrimal duct. Although most eyedrops are well tolerated by patients they can be associated with severe systemic side-effects resulting from absorption through the mucous membrane of the nasolacrimal duct. The risk of these side effects can be decreased by reducing the size of the eyedrop from the normal commercial volume of 25 μl. Lynch (1988) has designed eyedropper tips that, by varying the relationship between the inner and outer diameters of the end of the tip, are capable of delivering a drop of 8-10 μl. The use of a smaller eyedropper results in a reduced systemic drug absorption.

Tear film dynamics are affected by systemically administered pharmacological agents and locally-applied adjuvants. Timolol applied topically reduces tear flow whereas pilocarpine stimulates tear flow. The adjuvant benzalkonium chloride disrupts the tear film whereas methylcellulose increases the stability of the tear film.

Lacrimal Drainage System
An efficient drainage system exists to remove excess lacrimal fluid and cell debris from the precorneal area of the eye (Figure 8.6). The drainage of tears takes place along the lacrimal passages which are lined by a mucous membrane. Tears initially drain through the lacrimal puncta which are small circular openings of the lacrimal canalculi situated on the medial aspect of both the upper and lower lid margins. The superior and inferior canaliculi (approximately 8 mm in length and 1 mm in diameter) unite in the region of the medial canthus to form the common canalculus. This opens into the lacrimal sac about 3 mm below its apex and at its lower end is continuous with the nasolacrimal duct which passes downwards to open into the inferior meatus of the nose with a valvular mechanism at its opening. The tears finally pass into the nasopharynx.

The drainage of tears is an active process involving the lacrimal pump which is

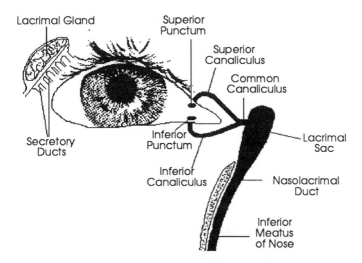

Figure 8.6. - The lacrimal drainage system

dependent on the integrity of the *orbicularis* muscle of the eyelids. Closure of the eyelids draws the lacrimal fluid from the puncta and canalculi into the sac by a suction effect, and the opening of the lids forces the lacrimal fluid from the sac into the nasolacrimal duct and then into the nose through the lower end of the sac. The valvular mechanism opens during this movement.

Blood-Eye Barriers
There are several tissues which act as blood-eye barriers in the ocular circulation. Topically applied fluorescein is seen to leak across the choroidal circulation, without passing through to the retinal pigment layer. The iris is a further barrier, since its blood vessels have thick walls which prevent leakage of materials into the aqueous humour. Ciliary epithelium in the ciliary processes is a unique membrane which prevents the passage of most molecules including antibiotics and proteins. However, molecules may enter the posterior chamber during the active secretion process that forms aqueous humour. The blood-eye barriers can be damaged by injury or inflammation. The capillary endothelial and ciliary epithelial cells separate from each other in this case, resulting in destruction of the intercellular barrier and leakage of material (Smelser and Pei, 1965).

THE MECHANISM OF DRUG PERMEATION
The sequential barriers of epithelium, endothelium and stroma pose difficulties for drug absorption through the cornea. The epithelial and endothelial cells are rich in lipids and are mostly permeable to fat soluble substances, whereas the stroma is acellular with a high water content, making it permeable to water soluble substances. Therefore, to penetrate the intact cornea, a substance must be both water soluble and fat soluble. This is analogous to the transdermal absorption of drugs, where sequential hydrophobic and hydrophilic barriers are also found. The main consequence of this is that well absorbed drugs are those which have a mixed hydrophilic/hydrophobic nature with an intermediate partition coefficient.

The movement of water-soluble drugs through the stroma is rapid, and since the endothelium is not rate limiting, the stroma can be considered with the aqueous humour as a single barrier. Both the epithelium and the aqueous tissues can act as drug reservoirs; the hydrophilic stroma serves as a depot for water-soluble compounds such as catecholamines and their metabolites whereas the epithelium is the main depot for lipophilic molecules such as chloramphenicol (Mindel *et al.*, 1984).

For ionizable drugs, the unionized form will more easily penetrate the epithelium and endothelium. The trans-stromal route is preferred by the ionized form. Pilocarpine, a weak base, is an example of a drug whose ionization behaviour can be exploited to optimize its absorption. In pharmaceutical products, it is buffered at low pH for stability reasons, and consequently it is administered in an ionized (protonated) form. The eye drop solution should be only weakly buffered, thereby allowing the buffer capacity of tears to adjust the pH to the physiological range as rapidly as possible after instillation, converting the drug to the unionized form and allowing its transport across the hydrophobic epithelium. A rapid adjustment to physiological pH also decreases induced blinking and lacrimation.

Protein Binding
Estimates of the total protein content of tears range from 0.6 to 2% w/v, major fractions consisting of albumin, globulin and lysozyme. Drugs bound to the protein in the tear fluid may not permeate the cornea due to the additional bulk of the protein molecule; also protein binding of drugs to conjunctival tissues competes for the drug available for corneal absorption. Binding increases in certain disease states, particularly inflammatory conditions, due to higher secretion of proteins in tissue exudate.

The effect of protein binding on drug bioavailability has been demonstrated in the rabbit. The response to pilocarpine was measured after adding increasing amounts of rabbit serum albumin to the drug solutions prior to administration (Mikkelson *et al.*, 1973). A marked reduction in pupillary response was observed by the addition of 3% albumin, corresponding to a 75 - 100 fold reduction in applied drug, as calculated from pilocarpine dose-response curves. Loss of the available drug through protein binding can be minimized through the use of competitive inhibitors for the protein binding sites. For example, the presence of a suitable concentration of acetylpyridinium chloride increases the biological response to pilocarpine by a factor of ten since it competes for protein binding sites, increasing the concentration of free pilocarpine (Mikkelson *et al.*, 1973).

Optimisation of instilled volume
The amount of drug reaching the anterior chamber of the eye is determined by the net result of two competing processes:
    (i) the rate of drug loss from the precorneal area.
    (ii) the rate of drug uptake by the cornea (Sieg and Robinson, 1976).
The rapid rate of tear turnover and efficient drainage in the eye profoundly affect the bioavailabilities of topically applied ophthalmic drugs. When an ophthalmic

solution, usually 30-50 μl in volume, is instilled into the lower fornix, the reflex blink can causes as much as 20 μl to spill over the lid margin onto the skin. The remainder of instilled drug is drained through the lacrimal drainage system and removal of the instilled solution continues until the total tear volume returns to the normal volume of 7 μl. As the precorneal volume of fluid (lacrimal and instilled) becomes smaller, the turnover rate of lacrimal fluid will have a greater influence on the residual drug concentration. Therefore, a larger instilled volume will maximize the penetration of ophthalmic drugs, but a larger proportion will be wasted through drainage. As much as 80% of the instilled volume drains into the systemic circulation (Shell, 1982), which can lead to toxicity problems particularly in geriatric and paediatric patients (Patton and Francoeur, 1978; File and Patton, 1980). Chrai (1973) determined that a volume of 5-10 μl was optimum as it minimized side effects due to systemic absorption via the drainage apparatus. However, delivery devices which can reproducibly deliver such small volumes of solution are not yet commercially viable.

Once the drug penetrates the cornea and enters the aqueous humour it is distributed to all the internal tissues of the eye. The anterior chamber is in contact with the cornea, iris, ciliary body, lens and vitreous humour. The drug is rapidly distributed to these tissues and concentrations mirror those of the aqueous humour.

Pigmentation and drug effects
The intraocular distribution of drug differs in pigmented eyes. Lee and Robinson (1982) demonstrated a ten-fold increase in pilocarpine deposition in the iris-ciliary body of the pigmented rabbit eye compared with albinos, although the pilocarpine concentration in the aqueous humour was indistinguishable between the two. Pilocarpine is metabolised by tissue esterases and esterase activity is highest in the iris and ciliary body, followed by the cornea and aqueous humour (Lee, 1983). In the pigmented eyes, the pharmacological effect was reduced owing to a higher amount of esterase activity in the cornea and iris-ciliary body.

Drug Penetration Through The Sclera And Conjunctiva
Instilled drugs may be absorbed by the conjunctiva or other tissues and are therefore unavailable for corneal permeation. Drug absorbed by the conjunctiva is transported from the eye to the systemic circulation (Patton, 1980; Lee and Robinson, 1979). However, it has been shown that the non-corneal absorption route may contribute significantly to bioavailability for drugs such as timolol and inulin (Ahmed and Patton, 1984). Vasodilating drugs such as pilocarpine accelerate loss of coadministered drugs by their action on the conjunctival vessels (Lee and Robinson, 1979).

Drug penetration across the sclera, which is composed primarily of collagen and mucopolysaccharide, may constitute an important route for some drugs, particularly those with low corneal permeation. Drugs may diffuse across the sclera by three possible pathways:-
(1) through perivascular spaces

(2) through the aqueous media of gel-like mucopolysaccharides
(3) across the scleral substance, composed of a matrix of collagen fibrils.

An *in vitro* study using isolated corneal and scleral membranes of the rabbit has shown that scleral permeability was significantly higher than the respective corneal permeability for all the tested compounds (Ahmed *et al.*, 1987). The permeability coefficients were in the order propranolol > penbutolol > timolol > nadolol for the cornea and penbutolol > propranolol > timolol > nadolol for the sclera. It was suggested that the mechanism for scleral permeation was diffusion across the intercellular aqueous media, as in the case of the structurally similar corneal stroma. This mechanism alone however, cannot explain the substantially higher permeability of penbutolol and propranolol compared with the other compounds of similar molecular weight. A partitioning mechanism may account for these observations.

Drug administered to the posterior part of the eye is removed efficiently by diffusion into the circulation, and escapes through the canal of Schlemm, the route through which aqueous humour leaves the eye. From the canal of Schlemm, the drug leaves the eye through the veins penetrating the sclera. For this reason, drugs instilled topically do not reach therapeutic concentrations in the posterior part of the eye, and direct injection is the preferred method of administration.

FACTORS INFLUENCING DRUG RETENTION
Osmolarity
The osmolarity of tears is directly proportional to the number of dissolved ions and non-ionizing solutes. Due to their molecular weight and low concentrations, proteins contribute only slightly to the total osmotic pressure (Van Ooteghem, 1987). The tonicity of human tears is influenced by the evaporation process when the eye is open. The osmolarity after prolonged eye closure or during sleep is 293 to 288 mOsm Kg^{-1} (Terry and Hill, 1978). After the eye is opened, the osmolarity varies from 302 to 318 mOsm Kg^{-1} (Gilbard and Farris, 1978; Farris *et al.*, 1981; Terry and Hill 1978). During the day, the osmolarity progressively rises at a rate of 1.43 mOsm Kg^{-1} hr^{-1} (Benjamin and Hill, 1983).

When an ophthalmic formulation is instilled into the eye, it mixes with the precorneal tear film. The osmotic pressure of the mixture depends upon the osmolarity of the tears and of the ophthalmic formulation. If the osmotic pressure obtained is within defined limits (Table 8.1), no discomfort is experienced, but if the osmotic pressure is outside these limits the patient experiences irritation eliciting reflex tears and blinking. The original osmolarity of the precorneal tear film is regained two minutes after the non-isotonic solution is administered (Holly and Lamberts, 1981), mainly due to a rapid flow of water across the cornea (Mishima, 1965). The instillation of a hypotonic drug solution creates an osmotic gradient between the tear film and the surrounding tissues, which induces a flow of water from the eye surface to the cornea, increasing temporarily the drug concentration on the eye surface (Bardendsen *et al.*, 1979).

Table 8.1. - Osmolarities of ophthalmic formulations provoking discomfort or irritation
(from Van Ooteghem, 1987)

Osmolarity (mOsm/Kg)	Authors
<100	Bisantis *et al.*, (1982)
<266	Riegelmann and Vaughan (1958)
	Trolle Lassen (1958)
>455	Trolle Lassen (1958)
>480	Riegelmann and Vaughan (1958)
>640	Maurice (1971)
	Bisantis *et al.*, (1982)

pH

The normal pH of tears varies between 7.0 and 7.4. Solutions instilled into the lower fornix with pH below 6.6 and above 9.0 are associated with irritation, reflex tears and blinking (Martin and Mims, 1950). The pH of the tear film is influence by the dissolved substances, some of which form buffer systems, for example bicarbonate-carbon dioxide.

When the eyelids are open, the pH of the precorneal tear film increases through loss of carbon dioxide. After an ophthalmic formulation is instilled into the eye, it is mixed with the tears present in the conjunctival sac and with the precorneal tear film. The pH of the mixture is mainly determined by the pH of the instilled solution. The tears have a very limited buffer capacity and since only the superficial layer of the tear film is eliminated by the movement of the eyelids, return to physiologically normal pH takes several minutes (Norn, 1985).

Viscosity

The viscosity of tears is influenced by proteins dissolved in the lacrimal fluid. The viscosity of human tears ranges from 1.3 to 5.9 mPa.s with a mean value of 2.916 mPa.s (Schuller *et al.*, 1972). The viscosity of ophthalmic solutions is often increased in order to obtain longer retention of a drug on the corneal surface. However, the instillation of viscous solutions can cause irritation, and solutions which become so thick that they require a force of more than approximately 0.9 N to shear them markedly interfere with blinking.

Preservatives

Nearly all artificial tear solutions are multi-component mixtures that invariably contain preservatives. At high concentrations, preservatives can cause irritation and damage to the ocular surface. Benzalkonium chloride is probably one of the most damaging preservatives. In strengths greater than 0.01 percent it can damage the corneal epithelium by desquamation. Disruption of the corneal barrier by benzalkonium chloride increases the ocular absorption non-selectively of several compounds of differing water solubility and molecular weight (Pfister and Burstein, 1976).

Effect of systemically-administered drugs

Certain drugs influence the tear secretion and/or blink frequency; for example, general anaesthetics may completely inhibit lid movements (Dundee *et al.*, 1982). When an ophthalmic formulation is to be prescribed it is important to know which other drugs are used by the patient. Antihypertensives administered systemically (e.g. reserpine, diazoxide) stimulate tear flow whilst antihistamines reduce tear flow.

ROUTES OF DRUG ADMINISTRATION

There are three main routes commonly used for administering drugs to the eye:
(a) Topical - drops or ointment
(b) Systemic - oral or injection
(c) Intra-ocular injection

Topical Administration

Drops

The most common form of topical administration is the eye drop which is easy to use, relatively inexpensive and does not impair vision. The major problem with this type of formulation is its inability to sustain high local concentrations of drug. Most eye-drops consist of an aqueous medium, to which can be added buffers (phosphate, borate, acetate and glucuronate), organic and inorganic excipients, emulsifiers, and wetting agents in order to accommodate a wide range of drugs with varying degrees of polarity. Vehicles may include water, aqueous mixtures of lower alkanols, vegetable oils, polyalkylene glycols, petrolatum based jelly, ethylcellulose, ethyl oleate, carboxymethylcellulose and polyvinylpyrrolidone. Aqueous eye-drops allow only a short duration of drug action, but the contact time between the vehicle and the eye can be increased by the addition of polymers such as polyvinyl alcohol and methylcellulose, although generally the effects on drug absorption are undramatic.

Sprays

Spray systems produce similar results to eye-drops in terms of duration of drug action and side-effects and can be produced in various concentrations. Sprays have several advantages over eye-drops: a more uniform spread of drug can be achieved and precise instillation requires less manual dexterity than the use of eye-drops. Contamination and eye injury due to eye-drop application are avoided and spray delivery causes less reflex lacrimation. A spray is particularly useful for treating patients whose hand movements are unsteady. The only disadvantage is that sprays are more expensive to produce than eye-drops so they are not as widely used.

Perfusion

Continuous and constant perfusion of the eye with drug solutions can be achieved by the use of ambulatory motor driven syringes which deliver drug solutions through fine polyethylene tubing positioned in the conjunctival sac. The flow rate of the perfusate through a minipump can be adjusted to produce continuous irrigation of the eye surface (3 to 6 ml min^{-1}) or slow delivery (0.2 ml min^{-1}) to avoid overflow (Ralph *et al.*, 1975). This system allows the use of a lower drug concentration than used in conventional eye-drops, yet will produce the same potency. Side effects are reduced and constant therapeutic action is maintained (Birmingham *et al.*, 1976). This system is not used very often due to the inconvenience and the cost involved, but may find application for drugs which are irritant and which have to be administered in sight-threatening situations.

Ointments

Ointments are also used, but are not as popular as eye drops since vision is blurred due to the oil base, making ointments impractical for day-time use. They are usually applied overnight or if the eye is to be bandaged. They are especially useful for paediatric use since small children often wash out drugs by crying. Ointments are generally nontoxic and safe to use on the exterior of the eye; however, ointment bases such as lanolin, petrolatum and vegetable oil are toxic to the interior of the eye, causing corneal edema, vascularization, scarring and endothelial damage (Scheie *et al.*, 1965). Intraocular contamination with these vehicles should therefore be avoided.

Ointments are used to prolong the contact time and thus increase the amount of drug absorbed. Hardberger and coworkers (1975) found that the half-time for the corneal clearance of a white petrolatum-mineral oil ointment was 35 minutes in the rabbit and 9.7 minutes in man. Two possible explanations for their longer retention were suggested; firstly, the bases are large viscous molecules which are not easily removed by blinking, and secondly, the oil bases are similar in nature to the superficial layer of the precorneal tear film and hence mix and are retained by the tear film. Antibiotics such as tetracyclines are used in the form of an ointment, producing effective antibacterial concentrations in the anterior chamber for several hours (Hardberger *et al.*, 1975), whereas an aqueous solution of tetracycline is ineffective for intraocular infections.

A problem with extremely lipophilic drugs, including corticosteroids, is that the therapeutic agent may partition into the oil base and not be released. For these drugs, alternative systems such as water soluble inserts may be preferable.

Particulates

Particulate carriers have been used to increase the duration of drug action. Formulations of 2% w/v pilocarpine adsorbed onto a biocompatible latex of average size 0.3 µm maintained a constant miosis in the rabbit for up to 10 hours compared to 4 hours with pilocarpine eye drops (Gurny, 1981).

Gamma scintigraphic studies have shown that the corneal retention of a radiolabelled soluble marker can be increased by formulation in a pH-sensitive dispersion, a temperature-setting gel or a mucopolysaccharide such as hyaluronic acid (Gurny *et al.*, 1987; Wilson 1987). The precorneal clearance half-times of various ophthalmic preparations are shown in Figures 8.7a and 8.7b.

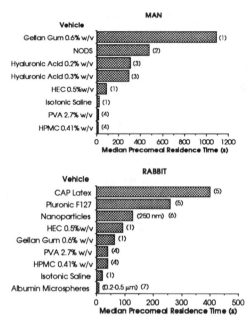

Figures 8.7a and b - The time for 50% clearance of various ophthalmic preparations from the corneal surface

(1) Greaves *et al.*, (1989). (2) Wilson *et al.*, (1989). (3) Snibson *et al.*, (1989). (4) Zaki *et al.*, (1986). (5) Gurny *et al.*, (1987). (6) Fitzgerald *et al.*, (1987). (7) Wilson *et al.*, (1983)

Sustained Release Devices

Provision of a matrix to sustain drug release in the eye can be achieved in several ways. For example, a hydrophilic (soft) contact lens can serve as a drug reservoir. The drug is incorporated into the lens in one of two ways, either by instilling drops on the lens when in place in the eye, or by presoaking the lens in a solution of the drug. Other systems are not placed on the cornea, but are inserted under the eyelid, such as insoluble inserts of polyvinyl alcohol or soluble collagen which dissolve in lacrimal fluid or disintegrate while releasing the drug. Soluble inserts are made of such substances as gelatin, alginates, agar and hydroxypropylmethylcellulose. These systems have been developed as a method for delivering larger amounts of drugs to the eye over a long period of time.

Ocuserts® (Alza Corporation, U.S.A.) are insoluble inserts containing pilocarpine used in the treatment of glaucoma, and have a one week duration of action. The major advantages of this system include longer duration of drug action, avoidance of accommodative spasms in younger patients and better patient compliance with the therapy (Chiou and Watanabe, 1982). However, 20% of all patients treated with the Ocusert® lose the device without being aware of the loss. For this reason, patients fitted with the device should be checked regularly.

The collagen shield made from porcine scleral tissue which is extracted and moulded into a contact lens-like configuration has proved useful as the basis of a drug delivery device. The shield conforms to the shape of the eye and lubricates the cornea as it dissolves. The dissolution time can be controlled to release over a period from approximately 12 hours to 72 hours and is related to the amount of cross-linkage produced by exposure to ultraviolet light during the manufacturing process. Drugs can be incorporated in the collagen matrix during manufacture, adsorbed into the shield during rehydration, or applied topically over the shield in the eye. As the shield dissolves, the drug is released gradually into the tear film, maintaining high concentrations on the corneal surface and increasing drug permeation through the cornea (Shofner *et al.*, 1989). Experimental studies suggest that drug delivery by collagen shields may be helpful in the early management of bacterial keratitis, in preference to frequent administration of topical antibiotics, subconjunctival injection, or topical administration over a soft contact lens.

An ophthalmic delivery system based on PVA gel which hydrates on contact with eye has been evaluated in our laboratories (Wilson *et al.*, 1989). In normal subjects, the PVA gel is cleared from the eye with a mean half-life of 8 minutes. The system shows great promise for prolonged drug delivery since vision is not affected by the presence of an insert positioned on the sclera.

Systemic Administration

Drugs are usually administered systemically for the treatment of diseases involving the optic nerve, retina and uveal tract. The blood/aqueous barrier only allows drugs to pass into the anterior chamber of the eye by one or two processes, both of which are very slow:
(1) secretion from the ciliary body
(2) diffusion from the capillaries of the iris.
Most drugs are unable to reach the anterior chamber in therapeutically active concentrations because either they are bound to plasma proteins and hence cannot pass through the blood vessel wall, or they are not sufficiently lipid soluble.

Some drugs such as acetazolamide are ineffective when given topically (Chiou and Watanabe, 1982). Acetazolamide can be administered parenterally but this is impractical for chronic drug administration. A delayed-release oral preparation of acetazolamide is valuable for patients with glaucoma since the sustained-release acetazolamide can maintain a more consistent level of drug for a longer period of time than the peaks and valleys attained with pulse injections.

Iontophoresis

Iontophoresis facilitates drug penetration through the intact corneal epithelium by electrically negating the charge of an ionized molecule by passage of a small current. The solution of the drug is kept in contact with the cornea in an eye-cup bearing an electrode. A potential difference is applied with the electrode in the cup having the same charge as the drug to repel it. This method of administration is very rarely used, except under carefully controlled conditions. Iontophoresis allows penetration of antibiotics that are ionized and therefore do not penetrate by other methods (for example, polymyxin B used in the local treatment of infections).

Intra-ocular Injection

Injections deliver larger quantities of drug more precisely into the eye. They have the disadvantage that it is a potentially painful route of administration. Repeated topical application of drugs can achieve the same results in most cases, and consequently, ocular injections are not used except in the last resort.

CONCLUSIONS

Increasing the residence time of an ophthalmic formulation on the corneal surface increases the drug bioavailability and therefore reduces frequency of administration. Although recent advances have been made in ocular drug delivery systems, eye drops are still the most commonly used formulations as they are the least expensive preparations, are easy to use, and do not interfere with vision. However, frequent administration is necessary.

The retention of a drug on the corneal surface is determined by the amount of tear flow and by the blink frequency, which can be stimulated by different factors. The most important factor influencing the retention of a drug on the corneal surface appears to be the properties of the drug itself. If a drug irritates the eye, it is difficult to obtain a long retention, but if the drug is non-irritant, retention time can be increased by instillation of small drops, by adjustment of the osmolarity, tonicity, pH and by choosing the appropriate preservatives and adjuvants.

REFERENCES

Ahmed I. and Patton T.F. (1984) Effect of pH and buffer on the precorneal disposition and ocular penetration of pilocarpine in rabbits. *Int. J. Pharmaceut.* **19** 215-218.

Ahmed I., Gokhale R.D., Shah M.V. and Patton T.F. (1987) Physicochemical determinants of drug diffusion across the conjunctiva, sclera and cornea. *J. Pharm. Sci.* **26** 583-586.

Barendsen H., Oosterhuis J.A. and Van Haeringen N.J. (1979) Concentration of fluorescein in tear fluid after instillation as eye drops: II. Hypotonic eye drops. *Ophthalmic Res.* **11** 83-89.

Benjamin W.J. and Hill R.M. (1983) Human tears: osmotic characteristics. *Invest. Ophthalmol. Vis. Sci.* **24** 1624-1626.

Birmingham A.T., Galloway N.R., Spencer S.A. and Walker D.A. (1976) Continuous infusion of the conjunctival sac with pilocarpine in normal subjects and in patients with chronic glaucoma. *Trans. Ophthal. Soc. U.K.* **96** 322-324.

Bisantis C., Squeri C.A., Colsi P., Provenzano P. and Trombetta C. (1982) Sur l'usage des collyres hypo-, iso- et hyper-osmotiques, acides ou alcalins, dans le dianostic et le traitement des anomalies de la secretion des larmes. *Bull. Memoir. Soc. Fran. Ophthalmol.* **94** 75-78.

Chiou G.C.Y. and Watanabe K. (1982) Drug delivery to the eye. *Pharmac. Ther.* **17** 269-278.

Chrai S.S., Patton T.F., Mehla A. and Robinson J.R. (1973) Lacrimal and instilled fluid dynamics in rabbit eyes. *J. Pharm. Sci.* **62** 1112-1121.

Dundee J.M., Hassard T.H., McGovan W.A. and Henshaw J. (1982) The "induction" dose of thiopentone. A method of study and preliminary illustrative results. *Anaesthesia* **37** 1176-1184.

Farris R.L., Stuchell R.N. and Mandel I.D. (1981) Basal and reflex human tear analysis. I Physical measurements: osmolarity, basal volumes and reflex flow rate. *Ophthalmology* **88** 852-857.

File R.R. and Patton T.F. (1980) Topically applied pilocarpine. Human pupillary response as a function of drop size. *Arch. Ophthalmol.* **98** 112-115.

Fitzgerald P., Hadgraft J., Kreuter J. and Wilson C.G. (1987) A gamma scintigraphic evaluation of microparticulate ophthalmic delivery systems: liposomes and nanoparticles. *Int. J. Pharm.aceut* **40** 81-84.

Gilbard P.J. and Farris R.L. (1978) Osmolarity of tear microvolumes in keratoconjunctivitis sicca. *Arch. Ophthalmol.* **96** 677-681.

Greaves J.L., Wilson C.G., Rozier A., Grove J. and Plazonnet B. (1989) Scintigraphic assessment of an ophthalmic gelling vehicle in man and rabbit. in preparation.

Gurny R. (1981) Preliminary study of prolonged acting "drug" delivery system for the treatment of glaucoma. *Pharm. Acta. Helv.* **56** 130-132.

Gurny R., Ibrahim H., Aebi A., Buri P., Wilson C.G., Washington N., Edman P. and Camber O. (1987) Design and evaluation of controlled release systems for the eye. *J. Controlled Release* **6** 367-373.

Hardberger R.E., Hanna C. and Goodart R. (1975) Effects of drug vehicles on uptake of tetracycline. *Am. J. Ophthalmol.* **80** 133-138.

Holly F.J. and Lamberts D.W. (1981) Effect of non-isotonic solutions on tear film osmolarity. *Invest. Ophthalmol. Vis. Sci.* **20** 236-245.

Kayes J. and Holmberg A. (1960) The fine structure of Bowman's layer and the basement membrane of the corneal epithelium. *Am. J. Ophthalmol.* **50** 1013-1021.

Lee V.H.L. and Robinson J.R. (1979) Mechanistic and quantitative evaluation of precorneal pilocarpine disposition in albino rabbits. *J. Pharm. Sci.* **68** 673-683.

Lee V.H.L. and Robinson J.R. (1982) Disposition of pilocarpine in the pigmented rabbit eye. *Int. J. Pharmaceut.* **11** 155-165.

Lee V.H.L. (1983) Esterase activities in adult rabbit eyes. *J. Pharm. Sci.* **72** 239-244.

Ludwig A. and Van Ooteghem M.M. (1987) The influence of the osmolality on the precorneal retention of ophthalmic solutions. *J. Pharm. Belg.* **42** 259-266.

Lynch M.G. (1988) Reducing the size and toxicity of eye drops. Presented at the Tenth National Science Writers Seminar in Ophthalmology, Arlington, Virginia. 25th-28th September 1988. Eye Research Seminar.

Martin F.N. and Mims J.L. (1950) Preparation of ophthalmic solutions with special reference to hydrogen-ion concentration and tonicity. *Arch. Ophthalmol.* **44** 561.

Maurice D.M. (1971) The tonicity of an eye drop and its dilution by tears. *Exp. Eye Res.* **11** 30-33.

Maurice D.M. (1972) The location of the fluid pump in the cornea. *J. Physiol.* **221** 43-54.

Mikkelson T.J., Chrai S.S. and Robinson J.R. (1973) Altered bioavailability of drugs in the eye due to drug protein interaction. *J. Pharm. Sci.* **62** 1942-1945.

Mishima S. and Maurice D.M. (1961) The oily layer of the tear film and evaporation from the corneal surface. *Exp. Eye Res.* **1** 39-45.

Mishima S. (1965) Some physiological aspects of the precorneal tear film. *Arch. Ophthalmol.* **73** 233-241.

Norn M.S. (1985) Tear pH after instillation of buffer *in vivo*. *Acta. Ophthalmol.* **55** 23-24.

Patton T.F. (1980) Ocular drug disposition. in *Ophthalmic Drug Delivery Systems*. ed Robinson J.R. A.Ph.A. Academy of Pharmaceutical Sciences, Washington, pp 28-54.

Patton T.F. and Francoeur M. (1978) Ocular bioavailability and systemic loss of topically applied ophthalmic drugs. *Am. J. Ophthalmol.* **85** 225-229.

Pedler C. (1962) The fine structure of the corneal epithelium. *Exp. Eye. Res.* **1** 286-289.

Pfister R.R. and Burstein N.L. (1976) The effects of ophthalmic drugs, vehicles and preservatives on corneal epithelium: a scanning electron microscope study. *Invest. Ophtalmol. Vis. Sci.* **15** 246-259.

Ralph R.A., Doane M.G. and Dohlman C.H. (1975) Clinical experience with a mobile ocular perfusion pump. *Arch. Ophthalmol.* **93** 1039-1043.

Riegelman S. and Vaughan D.G. (1958) Ophthalmic solutions. *J. Am. Pharm. Ass., Pract. Ed.* **8** 474-477.

Scheie H.G., Rubenstein A. and Katowitz J.A. (1965) Ophthalmic ointment bases in the anterior chamber. *Arch. Ophthalmol.* **73** 36-42.

Schuller W.O., Yang W.H. and Hill R.M. (1972) Clinical measurements of tears. *J. Am.*

Optom. Ass. **43** 1358-1361.

Shell J.W. (1982) Pharmacokinetics of topically applied ophthalmic drugs. *Surv. Ophthalmol.* **26** 207-218.

Shofner R.S., Kaufman H.E. and Hill J.M. (1989) New horizons in ocular drug delivery. in *Ophthalmology Clinics of North America* Vol 2 - No 1. Zimmerman T.J. and Kooner K.S. W.B. Saunders Co., Philadelphia.

Sieg J.W. and Robinson J.R. (1976) Mechanistic studies on transcorneal permeation of pilocarpine. *J. Pharm. Sci.* **65** 1816-1822.

Smelser G.K. and Pei Y.F. (1965) Cytological basis of protein leakage into the eye following paracentesis. *Invest. Ophthalmol. Vis. Sci.* **4** 249-263.

Snibson G.R., Greaves J.L., Soper N.J.W., Prydal J.I., Wilson C.G. and Bron A.J. (1989) Precorneal residence times of sodium hyaluronate solutions studied by quantitative gamma scintigraphy. *Submitted to Eye*

Terry J.E. and Hill R.M. (1978) Human tear osmotic pressure. diurnal variations and the closed eye. *Arch Ophthalmol.* **96** 120-122.

Trolle-Lassen C. (1958) Investigations into the sensitivity of the human eye to hypo- and hypertonic solutions as well as solutions with unphysiological hydrogen ion concentrations. *Pharm. Weekbl.* **93** 148-155.

Van Ooteghem M.M. (1987) Factors influencing the retention of ophthalmic solutions on the eye surface. in *Ophthalmic Drug Delivery. Biopharmaceutical, Technolgical and Clinical Aspects.* ed. Saettone M.S., Gucci G. and Speiser P. Fidia Research Series, Vol 11, Liviana Press, Padova.

Wilson C.G., Olejnik O. and Hardy J.G. (1983) Precorneal drainage of polyvinyl alcohol solutions in the rabbit assessed by gamma scintigraphy. *J. Pharm. Pharmacol.* **35** 451-454.

Wilson C.G. (1987) Scintigraphic evaluation of polymeric formulations for ophthalmic use. in *Ophthalmic Drug Delivery. Biopharmaceutical, Technolgical and Clinical Aspects.* ed. Saettone M.S., Gucci G. and Speiser P. Fidia Research Series, Vol 11, Liviana Press, Padova.

Wilson C.G., Fitzgerald P., Gilbert D. and Hollingsbee D. (1989) Scintigraphic assessment of the ophthalmic clearance of a PVA gel insert in man. (in preparation).

Wolff E. (1946) Mucocutaneous junction of lid-margin and distribution of tear fluid. *Trans. Opthal. Soc. UK.* **66** 291-308.

Zaki I., Fitzgerald P., Hardy J.G. and Wilson C.G. (1986) A comparison of the effect of viscosity on the precorneal residence of solutions in man and rabbit. *J. Pharm. Pharmacol.* **38** 463-466.

9

Nasal Drug Delivery

The nasal cavity is an irregularly-shaped space in the front of the head extending from the bony palate upwards to the cranium (Figure 9.1). It is bisected into the right and left cavities by the nasal septum and the front of each cavity opens onto the face through the nostrils. The back opens into the nasopharynx and then into the the trachea or oesophagus. The function of the nasal cavity is to filter, humidify and warm inspired air. The hairs at the nostril entrance and the cilia of the epithelium filter particles entering the nose. The mucosal lining of the nasal cavity also entraps particles by impingement and sedimentation. Warming and humidification is provided by the narrow passageways of the upper respiratory tract which have a good blood supply and transfer heat and water vapour to inhaled air. The upper portion of the middle cavity is the olfactory region containing receptors for smell.

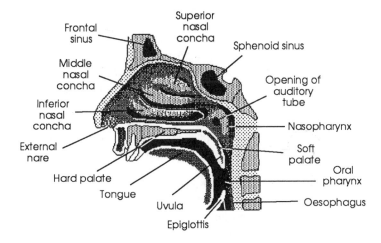

Figure 9.1. - Anatomy of the nasal cavity

Intranasal drug delivery is generally employed for topical action of drugs to treat allergies and infections which cause nasal irritation, sneezing and congestion. Although sympathomimetics used as nasal decongestants and antihistamines are used for their local action, these drugs have been shown to have systemic effects, suggesting that the nasal route can be an effective absorption pathway. This observation has encouraged research on delivery of large molecules, including peptides and proteins, via this route.

ANATOMY AND PHYSIOLOGY OF THE NASAL PASSAGES

The bony framework of the nasal cavity is formed by the fusion of seven bones (Figure 9.2). The nasal cavity is a chamber approximately 7.5 cm long by 5 cm high subdivided into the right and left halves by the nasal septum (Figure 9.3). The septum consists of the vomer and perpendicular plate of the ethmoid bone posteriorly, and the septal cartilage anteriorly, and terminates at the nasopharynx.

The two halves open to the front of the head through the anterior nasal apertures, the nares, whose diameter is controlled by the ciliator and compressor nares muscles and the *levator labii superioris alaeque* muscle. The entrance of the nares is guarded by hairs (vibrissae). The mean cross-sectional area of each nostril is 0.75 cm^2. The posterior nasal apertures, the *choanae*, link the nose with the rhinopharynx, are much larger than the nares and measure approximately 2.5 cm high by 1.2 cm wide (Hilding, 1963).

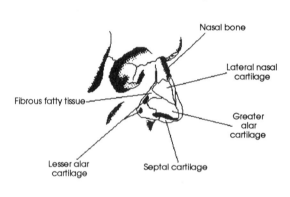

Nasal bone

Lateral nasal cartilage

Fibrous fatty tissue

Greater alar cartilage

Lesser alar cartilage   Septal cartilage

Figure 9.2. - Bony structure of the nose

The nasal cavity widens in the middle and is approximately triangular in shape. Most of the space is filled by obstructing vanes, the superior, middle and inferior turbinates or nasal conchae which form flues through which the air flows. The flues are quite narrow and cause the air to flow in such a way that no part of the airstream is very far from the moist mucous blanket lining the air spaces. The turbulent airflow through this region and the changes in direction caused by the turbinates encourages inertial impaction of suspended particles. The width of the air spaces is adjusted by swell bodies in the septum and turbinates.

Each half of the nasal cavity is composed of three parts: the nasal vestibule limited above and behind by the internal ostium, the olfactory region localised near to the superior turbinate and the opposite part of the septum, and the respiratory region comprising of the remainder of the cavity.

Heating and humidification of inhaled air are important functions of the nose which are facilitated by the abundant blood flow through the arteriovenous anastomoses in the turbinates. The rapid blood flow through the the *cavernous sinusoids* matches the cross-section of the nasal cavity to meet changing demands. Humidification is produced by an abundant fluid supply from the anterior serous glands, seromucous glands, goblet cells and by transudation (Mygind, 1979).

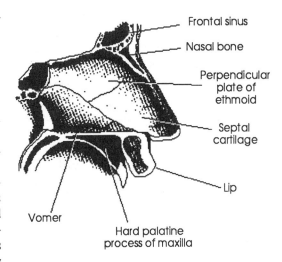

Figure 9.3. - Cross-section through the nose

Air can be brought to within 97 to 98% saturation, and inspired ambient air between -20°C and +55°C can be brought to within 10 degrees of body temperature.

The majority of the air flow from the nose to the pharynx passes through the middle meatus; however, up to 20% is directed vertically by the internal ostium to the olfactory region from where the airstream arches down to the nasopharynx. The sense of smell, olfaction, is performed by the olfactory cells of the nasal epithelial lining. These cells possess olfactory hairs, which when stimulated cause a receptor potential in the cell initiating a nerve impulse in the olfactory nerves to the brain.

Inhalation of irritants or allergens through the nose causes the subject to sneeze, which is a protective manoeuvre to expel the offending material. The sneeze reflex is similar to the cough reflex except that it applies to the nasal passages rather than the lower respiratory airways. During a sneeze, the uvula is depressed to channel the air through the nose and mouth to help clear the nasal passages of the irritation.

Nasal Epithelia
Over 60% of the epithelial surface of the nasopharyngeal mucosa is lined by stratified squamous epithelium. In the lateral walls and roof of the nasopharynx there are alternating patches of squamous and ciliated epithelia, separated by islets of transitional epithelium, which is also present in a narrow zone between the oropharynx and the nasopharynx. The lower area of the pharynx is lined with mucous membrane covered by stratified squamous epithelium. The posterior two-thirds of the nasal cavity is lined by pseudostratified epithelium possessing microvilli. These, along with the cilia, prevent drying of the surface and promote transport of water and other substances between the cells and the nasal secretions. The whole of the respiratory region is covered with goblet cells, which are

unicellular mucous glands and supply the surface with viscid mucus (Mygind, 1979).

The mucosal lining of the nasal cavity varies in thickness and vascularity. The respiratory region, which lines the majority of the cavity, is highly vascular and the surface of some of the epithelial cell types are covered in microvilli, increasing the area available for drug absorption.

Nasal Lymphatic System

The nasopharyngeal region possess a very rich lymphatic plexus, in which the lymph drains into deep cervical lymphatics. Besides capillary filtrate, some cerebrospinal fluid also drains into the nasal submucosa which is partly absorbed by the nasal lymphatics. When the nasal mucosa is damaged by an irritant, the resulting oedema results in an increased flow of lymph.

The lymphatics of the nasopharynx play an important part in the absorption of substances and particles which have been deposited on the nasal mucosa. Many materials, such as water, sodium chloride, prussian blue, phenolsulphophthalein, potassium iodide and pituitary hormone have been found to penetrate this region of the nasal mucosa. It is believed that these molecules diffuse mainly through the olfactory region of the mucosa to be taken up by the blood capillaries and to a lesser extent by the lymphatics.

Nasal Mucus

Mucus consists of mucopolysaccharides complexed with sialic acid and may be partially sulphated particularly in diseased conditions. The main component of mucus is water with 2 to 3% mucin and 1 to 2% electrolytes. Nasal mucus contains lysozymes, lactoferrin, interferon and antibodies to act on the filtered bacterial particles which become trapped in the mucus lining. Airborne particles of 2 to 4 μm diameter can penetrate into the lungs, but virus containing droplets often coalesce to exceed 5 to 6 μm in diameter and are therefore retained by the nose (Proctor *et al.*, 1973).

Mucociliary Clearance

Measurement

Many methods have been used to investigate nasal mucociliary clearance including direct observation, saccharin, radiological and gamma scintigraphic techniques. Bang and coworkers (1967) used sky blue dye to measure clearance rates and Andersen and coworkers (1971, 1974) used a saccharin test in which small amounts of the powder were placed in the nose and the transport measured as the time between application and detection of the taste. Puchelle and coworkers (1981) used aluminium discs of different colours which were placed on the floor and septum of the right and left nostril to measure transit rates in smokers and non-smokers. Quinlan and coworkers (1969) measured mucus flow rates using technetium-99m labelled "Amberlite" resin.

The average mucus flow rate is approximately 5 mm min^{-1} with a range from 0 to 20 mm min^{-1} (Andersen *et al.*, 1971; Proctor *et al.*, 1973). Although Andersen and coworkers (1972) found that the mucus flow in the anterior and posterior halves of the nasal cavity was identical, Quinlan and coworkers (1969) found that the transit rate tended to increase in the posterior portion, possibly due to less drying of the posterior mucosal surface by the stream of inspired air. The mean velocity of mucus flow and particle transport in the trachea is 14 mm min^{-1}, whereas in the upper bronchial tree and the lower bronchial tree and parenchyma, the rates are 1 and 0.5 mm min^{-1} respectively, i.e the mucus flow rate decreases towards the lungs (Morrow *et al.*, 1967).

There are differing opinions as to the effect of relative humidity on nasal mucociliary clearance. Studies by Ewert (1965), Quinlan and coworkers (1969) and Aoki and Crowley (1976) suggest that flow rate is correlated with relative humidity and that it increases from 6 to 9 mm min^{-1} when the relative humidity rises above 30%. However other studies have not observed significant differences in mucus flow or in nasal airway resistance at relative humidities ranging from 10 to 70% with similar temperatures to the previous studies of about 23ºC (Andersen *et al.*, 1972; Proctor *et al.*,1973; Andersen *et al.*, 1974; Proctor, 1983).

Irritants and particulates
There is a very wide normal range of mucociliary clearance which can be observed when particulates are introduced into the nose. Some people display the expected rapid, uninterrupted particle movement, whereas others have a slowing or even a halt in particle movement after an initial fast flow, or constantly slow movement or stasis (Andersen *et al.*, 1971). A constitutional element in the overall control of nasal mucociliary flow may exist, but the mucus flow rate may also be influenced by many environmental factors (Andersen *et al.*, 1974).

Bang and coworkers (1967) found no change in mucociliary clearance after exposure to increased temperature, smog, nasally exhaled cigarette smoke, clouds of dust or after mild dehydration. However nasal flushing or drinking very hot tea doubled the flow rate. Studies in rats have shown that inhalation of sulphur dioxide increases the thickness of the mucus blanket, and exposure to ammonia, formaldehyde and sulphur dioxide results in the cessation of ciliary movement to varying degrees (Dalhamn, 1956). The effect of irritants such as sulphur dioxide was greatest on the mucociliary transport in the anterior part of the nose, and for subjects with an initially slow mucus flow rate (Andersen *et al.*, 1974; Proctor, 1983).

Although Quinlan and coworkers (1969) and Puchelle and coworkers (1981) found no differences in transit rates for smokers and non-smokers, Ewert (1965) and Stanley and coworkers, (1986) found significantly longer nasal mucociliary clearance times in smokers (20.3 ± 9.3 minutes) compared to non-smokers (11.1 ± 3.8 minutes). However, the difference diminished at relative humidities greater than 45%. The defective clearance in smokers was thought to be due to a reduction in the number of cilia or a change in their viscoelastic properties rather than a slowing in cilia beat frequency.

It has been found that inhalation of wood dust impedes the normal mucociliary function of clearing the nasal mucous membranes and allows accumulation and retention of inhaled substances in the nasal cavity. The mucus transport rate decreases to less than 1 mm min^{-1} (mucostasis). It has been shown that the risk of developing adenocarcinoma of the nasal cavity and sinuses, especially the ethmoid, is enhanced in cabinetmakers and wood machinists in the furniture industry (Acheson *et al.*, 1968; Andersen *et al.*, 1976). It has also been found that individuals exposed to nickel may develop histological changes in nasal mucosa which can be precancerous (Torjussen and Solberg, 1976). Pathologies that affect mucus flow rates and therefore the clearance of nasal sprays may modify the efficacy of intranasally administered drugs.

Allergy

Hayfever is rhinoconjunctivitis due to pollen allergy. About 10% of the population are sufferers of this condition. Tickling in the nose, sneezing and watery rhinorrhea are the most troublesome symptoms but an intense itching of the soft palate can also be experienced indicating that the mucociliary system has transported allergenic substances to the rhinopharynx. The mucus clearance time will be decreased to between 3.3 and 5.6 minutes, because the nasal secretions become alkaline (pH 8.0) leading to an increase in ciliary activity (Hady *et al.*, 1983).

Perennial rhinitis can be defined as a disease giving rise to two or three of the following symptoms for over one hour on most days: sneezing attacks (greater than five sneezes), serous or seromucous hypersecretion, and nasal blockage due to a swollen nasal mucosa. There are three types of disease with similar symptoms but different aetiology. Allergic rhinitis is due to an allergen, the 'intrinsic' group shows eosinophilia and autonomic rhinitis which is probably caused by an auto-nomic imbalance. In all cases clearance rates are increased; in allergic rhinitis, this is due to alkaline nasal secretions causing an increase in ciliary activity, whereas in atrophic rhinitis, abnormal widening of nasal passages causes inspired air to push particles rapidly towards the nasopharynx (Hady *et al.*,1983).

Structural Dysfunction

Nasal polyps are round, soft, semi-translucent, yellow or pale glistening benign tumours usually attached to the nasal or sinus mucosa by a relatively narrow stalk or pedicle. Their presence prevents efficient humidification, temperature control and particle infiltration of inspired air. The nasal clearance is slowed down due to blockage of the nose and defects in ciliary action or mucous secretion (Figures 9.4 and 9.5) (Lee *et al.*, 1984). Eosinophil or allergic polyps are characterised by nasal eosinophilia, seromucous secretion and steroid responsiveness; whereas neutrophil or infectious polyps demonstrate nasal neutrophilia, purulent secretion and lack of effect of steroid treatment (Mygind, 1979).

Mucociliary flow rates are slowed down in Kartagener's syndrome (chronic

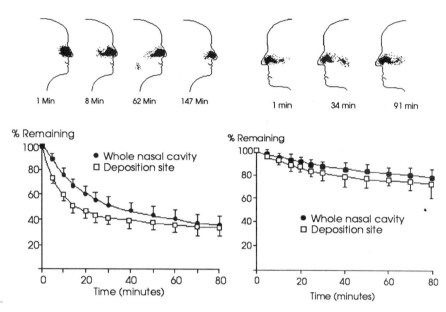

Figure 9.4. - Nasal spray deposition and clearance from the whole nasal cavity and deposition site in normals

Figure 9.5. - Nasal spray deposition and clearance from the whole nasal cavity and deposition site in patients prior to polypectomy

sinusitis, bronchiectasis, situs inversus) due to constant non-motility of cilia in the airways, probably caused by an inherited lack of dynein arms in the cilia (Pederson and Mygind, 1976).

Laryngectomies can affect nasal mucociliary clearance. Sakakura and coworkers (1983) found a significant acceleration in peak transport rate between patients with sixty days of laryngectomy in comparison to those patients who had had a laryngectomy greater than three years before. This could be partly due to a change in the nasal secretion.

Flow rates in twenty-four lepers who had differing degrees of nasal pathology indicated that, even with distortion, scarring or erosion of intranasal structures, any remaining intact mucosa which was protected from the direct impact of unmodified air functioned normally. However heavy crusting of mucous membranes was found to inhibit or prevent mucous flow (Bang *et al.*, 1967).

Infection
Hady and coworkers (1983) found that clearance times became faster (5.3 - 8.3 minutes) in cases of chronic sinusitis due to cilia functioning actively when bathed in pus, due to the increase in pH. They also found that people with deviated septa or rhinoscleroma had longer clearance times (25 - 35 minutes) than normal subjects (9 - 14.8 minutes). This was due to poor mucociliary transport due to obstruction, leading to an inspired air current concentrated on a restricted area of mucosa exceeding its capacity to saturate air. This caused an increase in the viscosity of the

nasal mucus, making it unsuitable for effective ciliary action.

Nasal mucociliary clearance rates change if a person is suffering from a cold. Clearance rates increased with copious mucous flow, but subjects recovering from a cold and experiencing nasal congestion had slower clearance times (Proctor *et al.*, 1973; Bond *et al.*, 1983). In a study at Nottingham nasal spray clearance was measured in a number of volunteers with colds. During mucus hypersecretion, less than 10% of the dose was found to remain in the nasal cavity after 25 minutes, whereas in the congested phase none of the dose had left the site of deposition 90 minutes after administration (Bond *et al.*, 1983). Subjects were not allowed to blow their noses during the investigation. Sneezing and nose-blowing would no doubt be an important consideration when studying the bioavailability of systemically acting compounds delivered via the nasal cavity.

Drug and Toxin-induced Changes
Many drugs administered as nasal preparations can influence ciliary motility. Hermens and Merkus (1987) have reviewed this area. Their list of materials which are ciliotoxic includes anaesthetics (Van de Donk *et al.*, 1982), antihistamines, propranolol (Duchateau, 1987), and bile salts (Duchateau *et al.*, 1986a), while β-adrenergic and cholinergic drugs stimulated ciliary motility.

Dexamethasone nasal drops (used in the treatment of allergic rhinitis) may cause pathological changes leading to Cushing's syndrome. The drug acts by absorption through the nasal mucosa and partly through the intestinal mucosa after a portion of the dose is swallowed. This problem does not occur with the newer intranasal steroids (e.g. beclomethasone and flunisolide) which are less readily absorbed through the nasal mucosa, and are inactivated in the liver after gastrointestinal absorption (Kimmerle and Rolla, 1985). Sakethoo and coworkers (1978) found that the two α-adrenergic nasal decongestant sprays, phenylephrine and tetrahydrozoline, often used in the management of allergic rhinitis, significantly increased nasal mucous velocity within ten minutes of administration. This is related to vasoconstriction of nasal mucosal vessels leading to a decrease in the fluid content of the mucosa. However, contrary to early *in vitro* studies which showed an inhibitory effect on ciliary function, Vinther and Elbrond (1978) found that penicillin administered orally did not alter ciliary action.

Much interest has been shown in the ciliotoxicity of formulation excipients included in nasal sprays. Van de Donk and Mercus (1981) reported that mercury-containing preservatives, e.g. thiomersal, should not be employed in nasal preparations since these materials produce a rapid, irreversible inactivation of cilia in a chick tracheal preparation. However Bond and coworkers (1983) showed that thiomersal present at concentrations used in these experiments had no effect on mucociliary transport in man.

ADMINISTRATION OF DRUGS INTRANASALLY
The intranasal route is very useful for avoiding injections in the young and is a good

way of administering drugs to the elderly. Many drugs can be given via the nasal route. However, the physiological conditions of the nose, i.e. vascularity, speed of mucus flow, retention and atmospheric conditions, will affect the efficacy of drugs or vaccines, as will the nature of the materials, e.g volume, concentration, density, viscosity, pH, tonicity, and pharmacological and immunological activity (Freestone and Weinberg, 1976; Stuart, 1973). The slower the clearance of the drug, the longer the time allowed for drug action or absorption.

Drugs

Drugs acting locally on the nose can be divided into three groups: i) those used in nasal allergy, ii) topical nasal decongestants and iii) anti-infective nasal preparations. The intranasal route has also been established as a suitable method of improving the systemic absorption of drugs which are subject to a significant gut wall and first-pass metabolism, those unstable in acid, and for polar compounds exhibiting poor oral absorption (Bond, 1987).

Drugs administered for local action

Symptomatic relief from the nasal congestion associated with vasomotor rhinitis, nasal polyps and the common cold can be obtained by short term use of decongestant nasal drops and sprays, for example ephedrine hydrochloride. Decongestants contain sympathomimetic drugs which exert their effect by vasoconstriction of the mucosal blood vessels which, in turn, reduce the thickness of the nasal mucosa. However, rebound vasodilation after administration of the vasoconstrictors phenylephrine and naphazoline (sympathomimetics) has been reported. This secondary vasodilatation produces a temporary increase in nasal congestion leading to further use of the decongestant (Snow *et al.*, 1980).

Drugs administered for systemic effect.

Drugs can be administered intranasally as an alternative to injection or if they are inactivated in the gastrointestinal tract. These include proteins, polypeptides, polar compounds, drugs subject to significant gut wall and first pass metabolism, or compounds possessing poor stability in gastrointestinal fluids (Freestone and Weinberg, 1976; Parr, 1983). Lignocaine is an example of one of these drugs, however it causes a highly significant increase in nasal width although it has no effect on nasal resistance to airflow (Jones, 1986). Drugs such as propranolol (Hussain *et al.*, 1979a,b, 1980), progesterone (Hussain *et al.*, 1981; David *et al.*, 1981) and enkephalins (Su *et al.*, 1985) appear to be absorbed effectively from the nasal route with bioavailabilities similar to that obtained for intravenous administration. Visor and co-workers (1986) found that nicardipine was well absorbed in a rat nasal model. Duchateau and co-workers (1986b) found that the hydrophilic drug metoprolol was well absorbed, but the hydrophobic alprenolol was poorly absorbed, compared to an oral dose, suggesting that hydrophobicity is important in determining nasal absorption. Ergotamine was poorly absorbed orally (5.1%), but well absorbed nasally (62%) (Hussain, 1984).

McMartin and coworkers (1987) have reviewed the absorption and availability of a wide range of nasally administered drugs, and correlated absorption with a range of molecular parameters such as hydrophobicity and molecular weight. They suggest that most small molecules are transported through hydrophobic channels between the cells which allow molecules up to 1000 Daltons to pass easily. This is consistent with the observed absorption of many peptides.

Peptides

The nasal mucosa possesses little metabolising capacity, unlike the gastrointestinal tract, and there have been several reports of efficient delivery of high and low molecular weight peptides via this route. Luteinising hormone releasing hormone (LHRH) and its analogues have been evaluated as potential contraceptive agents, although it has been shown that the dose employed has to be considerably higher that the parenteral dose (Berquist *et al.*, 1979). Human natriuretic peptide was effective in nasal doses of 0.5 to 0.6 μg (Shionoiri and Kaneko, 1986). Interferon was not absorbed in rabbits unless surfactants such as bile salts were coadministered (Maitani *et al.*, 1986) The nasal route is relatively unsuccessful for drugs such as insulin (Moses *et al.*, 1983; Salzman *et al.*, 1985), growth hormone releasing factor (Evans *et al.*, 1983) and calcitonin (Hanson et al., 1987), where bioavailability is low. Poor intranasal bioavailability of some peptides may be due to hydrolysis by peptidases present in nasal secretions (Hussain *et al.*, 1985) or simply due to limitations in the size of the hydrophilic pores through which they are thought to pass.

Surfactants

In rats, nasal absorption of polypeptides has been shown to be improved by co-administration with bile salts (Hirai *et al.*, 1981) and Su and coworkers (1985) demonstrated that the availability of an enkephalin analogue could be increased from 59% to 94% in this way. In a similar manner, insulin absorption has been shown to be improved by co-administration of sodium deoxycholate (Gordon *et al.*, 1985), and Moses and co-workers (1983) demonstrated an acceptable glucose-lowering response in human diabetics with a calculated bioavailability of between 10% and 30% of that of a parenteral dose. Similar encouraging results were reported by Paquot and co-workers (1988) using 0.25% Laureth-9 as the absorption-promoting agent. Co-administration of bile salts increases the absorption of the high molecular weight materials up to 6000 Daltons (Hersey and Jackson 1987; McMartin *et al.*, 1987). It was suggested that the mechanism involved was an action on junctional proteins which rendered the normally hydrophobic areas of contact hydrophilic. Since the use of these materials is associated with an interaction with the membrane causing a change in the epithelial structure, and the stasis of cilia, the long term use and safety of such materials as absorption enhancing adjuvants in the nose is questionable.

DRUG DELIVERY SYSTEMS AND DEPOSITION PATTERNS

The most popular delivery systems to the nasal mucosa are sprays and drops. A metered dose inhaler delivering a 0.1 ml dose with droplets of mean diameter 50 μm deposited anteriorly in the nasal cavity with little of the dose reaching the turbinates

(Bond *et al.*, 1983). Clearance was slow and predominantly progressed along the floor of the cavity. This may be compared with the pattern of deposition following nasal drops. A volume of around 90 µl applied nasally dispersed throughout the entire length of the cavity from atrium to nasopharynx (Hardy *et al.*, 1985) as shown in Figure 9.6. A single drop (30 µl volume) appeared to be insufficient to cover the nasal surface, but volumes larger than 100 µl had no effect on the extent of deposition and the excess material was swallowed (Aoki and Crawley, 1976). Bond and coworkers (1983) found that administration of a spray as one or two ejections had no apparent effect on the distribution. In all cases clearance followed a biphasic exponential pattern, with the second phase of clearance of spray being slower than drops. (Figure 9.7). A biphasic pattern has also been observed for the clearance of 0.25, 0.5 and 0.75 ml drops labelled by [^{99}Tc^m]-human serum albumin. The first phase appears to be due to the removal of the bulk of the

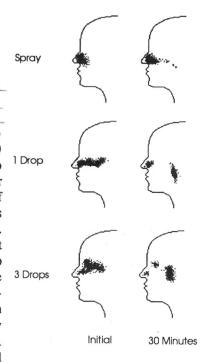

Figure 9.6. - Sites of deposition and patterns of clearance following adminstration of nasal spray and drops

activity, including boluses of material which break away from the deposition site due to traction of the mucus layer over the ciliated epithelia. Retention at the site of administration appears to be due to impaction of the spray formulation onto the non-ciliated vestibule and, since nose wiping or sneezing was discouraged, the material was slow to clear.

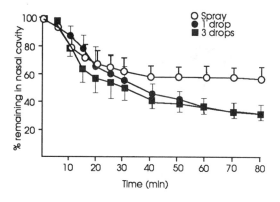

Figure 9.7. - Clearance from the nasal cavity of a spray and two volumes of drops

It has been found that hand-operated pumps for delivering aerosols require extensive priming before they produce a full dose, although a fairly reproducible dose is delivered from a metered dose freon-propelled pressurised aerosol. By valve selections, the manufacturer can adjust the volume of carrier gas per puff, but aerosols cannot deliver more than approximately 2 mg of active drug per puff. The distribution of drug produced is uneven with the anterior parts of the nasal cavity receiving the full impact of the aerosol (Mygind, 1979). Interestingly, during nasal breathing, aerosol sprays are retained in the nose and do not penetrate to the lower respiratory tract because 85 to 90% of the particulate matter has a diameter of greater than 5 to 6 μm (Ballenger, 1983), whereas 80 to 90% of droplets produced by nebulizers were cleared to the upper respiratory tract (Wolfsdorf *et al.*, 1969).

Vehicle Effects
It is well established that viscous solutions are cleared slowly from the eye and there has been some interest in the possibility of sustaining delivery to the nose by the incorporation of viscolysing agents in the formulation.

Pennington and coworkers (1988) compared the clearance of solutions thickened with 0.6 to 1.2% hydroxypropylmethylcellulose (HPMC) in man. This material demonstrates pseudoplastic behaviour at high concentrations, which is an advantage in a spray system since the material will shear-thin on activation of the pump but thicken on contact with the mucus layer. As shown in Figure 9.8, there was a clear relationship between the degree of thickening of the solution and the rate of clearance. Harris and coworkers (1988) used a similar technique to investigate the clearance of methylcellulose solutions at 0.25 and 0.5% compared with water, and noted a increase in particle size from 51 μm (0%), 81 μm (0.25%) to 200μm (0.5%). These authors found a biphasic pattern of clearance, with a slower clearance for the 0.25% methylcellulose than for water, but found that clearance of the 0.5% was faster than 0.25% solution.

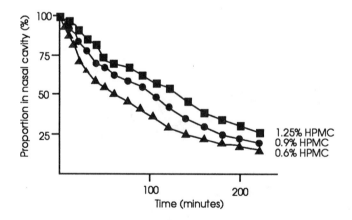

Figure 9.8. - Effect of HPMC on clearance of technetium-99m labelled diethylenetri-aminepentaacetic acid delivered by a nasal spray

lllum and co-workers (1987) have examined the clearance of various bioadhesive preparations for nasal drug delivery using microspheres composed of starch, diethylaminoethyl (DEAE) dextran and albumin labelled with technetium-99m. These were compared with powder and solutions of sodium cromoglycate labelled with technetium-99m diethylenetriaminepentaacetic acid (DTPA). Prolonged retention of DEAE dextran microspheres compared to the solutions was observed, due to impaction of the preparation onto the epithelium of the vestibular surfaces.

CONCLUSIONS

Drug delivery to the nasal cavity recently has received much interest for the delivery of proteins and peptides, but the results have been somewhat variable. Penetration enhancers improve bioavailability, but as their use in rectal delivery has shown, they make the membrane non-selectively "leaky", with the result that toxins can also enter the systemic circulation. The other major problem in using this route for the delivery of systemically acting compounds is that the common cold or hayfever will make residence time and hence drug absorption unpredictable.

REFERENCES

Acheson E.D., Cowdell R.H., Hadfield E. and Macbeth R.G. (1968) Nasal cancer in woodworkers in the furniture industry. *Br. Med. J.* **2** 587-596.

Andersen H.C., Solgaard J. and Andersen I. (1976) Nasal cancer and nasal mucus transport in woodworkers. *Acta Otolarnygol.* **52** 263-265.

Andersen I., Lundqvist G.R. and Proctor D.F. (1971) Human nasal mucosal function in a controlled climate. *Arch. Environ. Health* **23** 408-420.

Andersen I., Lundqvist G.R. and Proctor D.F. (1972) Human nasal function under four controlled humidities. *Am. Rev. Resp. Dis.* **106** 438-449.

Andersen I., Lundqvist G.R., Jensen P.L. and Proctor D.F. (1974) Human response to controlled levels of sulphur dioxide. *Arch. Environ. Health.* **28** 31-39.

Aoki F.K. and Crowley J.C.W. (1976) Distribution and removal of human serum albumin-technetium 99m instilled intranasally. *Br. J. Clin. Pharmacol.* **3** 869-878.

Ballenger J.J. (1983) Symposium: The nose versus the environment. *Laryngoscope* **93** 56-57.

Bang B.G., Mukherjee A.L. and Bang F.B. (1967) Human nasal mucous flow rates. *John Hopkins Med. J.* **121** 38-48.

Berquist C., Nillins S.J. and Wide L. (1979) Intranasal gonadotrophin-releasing hormone agonist as a contraceptive agent. *Lancet* **ii** 215-216.

Bond S.W., Hardy J.G. and Wilson C.G. (1983) Deposition and clearance of nasal sprays. *Proceedings of the 2nd European Congress of Biopharmaceutics and Pharmacokinetics*, Salamanca, Spain, pp93-97.

Bond S.W. (1987) Intranasal administration of drugs. In. *Drug Delivery to the Respiratory Tract.* ed Ganderton D. and Jones T.M. Ellis Horwood, Chicester. pp133-139.

Dalhamn T. (1956) Mucus flow and ciliary activity in the trachea of healthy rats and rats exposed to respiratory irritant gases. *Acta Physiol. Scand.* **36 Suppl. 123** 1-158.

David G.F.X., Puri C.P. and Anand Kumar T.C. (1981) Bioavailability of progesterone enhanced by intranasal spraying. *Experientia* **37** 533-534.

Duchateau G.S.M.J.E. (1987) Studies on nasal drug delivery. *Pharm. Weekblad* **9** 326-328.

Duchateau G.S.M.J.E., Zuidema J. and Merkus F.W.H.M. (1986a) Bile salts and intranasal drug absorption. *Int. J. Pharmaceut.* **31** 193-199.

Duchateau G.S.M.J.E., Zuidema J., Albers W.M. and Merkus F.W.H.M. (1986b) Nasal absorption of alprenolol and metoprolol. *Int. J. Pharmaceut.* **34** 131-136.

Evans W.S., Borges J.L.C., Kaiser D.L., Vance M.L., Seller R.P., Macleod R.M., Vale W., Rivier J. and Thorner M.O. (1983) Intranasal administration of human pancreatic tumor GH-releasing factor-40 stimulates GH release in normal men. *J. Clin. Endocrinol. Metab.* **57** 1081-1083.

Ewert G. (1965) On the mucus flow in the human nose. *Acta Otolaryngol. Suppl.* **200** 1-62.

Freestone D.S. and Weinberg A.L. (1976) The administration of drugs and vaccines by the nasal route. *Br. J. Clin. Pharmacol.* **3** 827-830.

Gordon G.S., Moses A.C., Silver R.D., Fleir J.S. and Carey M.C. (1985) Nasal absorption of insulin: Enhancement by hydrophobic bile salts. *Proc. Nat. Acad. Sci.* **82** 7419-7423.

Hady M.R., Shehata O. and Hassan R. (1983) Nasal mucociliary function in different diseases of the nose. *J. Laryngol. Otol.* **97** 497-501.

Hardy J.G., Lee S.W. and Wilson C.G. (1985) Intranasal drug delivery by spray and drop. *J. Pharm. Pharmacol.* **37** 294-297.

Hermens W.A.J.J. and Merkus F.W.H.M. (1984) The influence drugs on nasal ciliary movement. *Pharm. Res.* **4** 445-449.

Hersey S.J. and Jackson R.T. (1987) Effect of bile salts on nasal permeability in vitro. *J. Pharm. Sci.* **76** 876-879.

Hanson M., Gazdick G., Cahill J. and Augustine M. (1987) Intranasal delivery of the peptide, salmon calcitonin. In *Delivery Systems for Peptide Drugs* Ed. Davis S.S., Illum L. and Tomlinson E. Plenum, New York, pp 233-242.

Harris A.S., Svensson E., Wagner Z.G., Lethagen D. and Nilsson I.M. (1988). Effect of viscosity on particle size, deposition and clearance of nasal delivery systems containing desmopressin. *J. Pharm. Sci.* **77** 405-408.

Hilding A.C. (1963) Phagocytosis, mucous flow and ciliary action. *Arch. Environ. Health* **6** 61-71.

Hirai S., Yaskiki T. and Mima H. (1981) Mechanisms for the enhancement of the nasal absorption of insulin by surfactants. *Int. J. Pharmaceut.* **9** 173-184.

Hussain A., Hirai S. and Bawarshi R. (1979a) Nasal absorption of propranolol in rats. *J. Pharm. Sci.* **68** 1196.

Hussain A., Hirai S. and Bawarshi R. (1979b) Nasal absorption of propranolol from different dosage forms by rats and dogs. *J. Pharm. Sci.* **69** 1411-1413.

Hussain A., Hirai S. and Bawarshi R. (1981) Nasal absorption of the natural contraceptive steroid in rats - progesterone absorption (letter). *J. Pharm. Sci.* **70** 466-467.

Hussain A., Foster T., Hirai S., Kashihara T., Batenhorst R. and Jones M. (1980) Nasal absorption of propranolol in humans. *J. Pharm. Sci.* **69** 1240.

Hussain A., Kimura R., Huang C.H., and Mustafa R. (1984) Nasal absorption of ergotamine tartate in rats. *Int. J. Pharmaceut.* **21** 289-294.

Hussain A., Nassar R.B. and Huang C.H. (1985) in Transnasal systemic medications. Ed Chien Y.W. Elsevier, Amsterdam.

Illum L., Jorgensen H., Bisgaard H., Krogsgaard O. and Rossing N. (1987) Bioadhesive microspheres as a potential nasal drug delivery system. *Int. J. Pharmaceut.* **39** 189-199.

Jones A.S., Lancer J.M., Shone G. and Stevens J.C. (1986) The effect of lignocaine on nasal resistance and nasal sensation of airflow. *Acta Otolaryngol.* **101** 328-330.

Kimmerle R. and Rolla A.R. (1985) Iatrogenic Cushing's syndrome due to dexamethasone nasal drops. *Am. J. Med.* **79** 535-537.

Lee S.W., Hardy J.G. Wilson C.G., and Smelt G.J.C. (1984) Nasal sprays and polyps. *Nucl. Med. Commun.* **5** 697-703.

Maitani Y., Igawa T., Machida Y. and Nagai T. (1986) Intranasal administration of βinterferon in rabbits. *Drug Design and Delivery* **1** 65-70.

McMartin C., Hutchinson L.E., Hyde R. and Peters G.E. (1987) Analysis of structural requirements for the absorption of drugs and macromolecules from the nasal cavity. *J. Pharm. Sci.* **76** 535-540.

Morrow P.E., Gibb F.R. and Gazioglu K.M (1967) A study of particulate clearance from the human lung. *Am. Rev. Resp. Dis.* **96** 1209-1221.

Moses A.C., Gordon G.S., Carey M.C. and Flier J.S. (1983) Insulin administered intranasally as an insulin-bile salt aerosol: effectiveness and reproducibility in normal and diabetic subjects. *Diabetes* **32** 1040-1047.

Mygind N. (1979) Nasal Allergy. 2nd edition. Blackwell Scientific Publication, Oxford.

Paquot N., Scheen A.J., Franchimont P., Lefebvre P.J. (1988) The intra-nasal administration of insulin induces significant hypoglycaemia and classical counter-regulatory hormonal responses in normal man. *Diabetes Metab.* **14** 31-36.

Parr G.D. (1983) Nasal delivery of drugs. *Pharmacy International* **4** 202-205.

Pederson H. and Mygind N. (1976) Absence of axonemal arms in the nasal mucosa cilia in Kartagener's syndrome. *Nature* (London) **262** 494-495.

Pennington A.K., Ratcliffe J.H., Wilson C.G. and Hardy J.G. (1988) The influence of solution viscosity on nasal spray deposition and clearance. *Int. J. Pharm.* **43** 221-224.

Proctor D.F., Andersen I. and Lundqvist G. (1973) Clearance of inhaled particles from the human nose. *Arch. Intern. Med.* **131** 132-139.

Proctor D.F. (1983) Nasal mucus transport and our ambient air. *Laryngoscope* **93** 58-62.

Puchelle E., Aug F., Pham Q.T. and Bertand A. (1981) Comparison of three methods for measuring nasal mucociliary clearance in man. *Acta Otolaryngol.* **91** 297-303.

Quinlan M.F., Salman S.D., Swift D.L., Wagner H.N. and Proctor D.F. (1969) Measurement of mucociliary function in man. *Am. Rev. Resp. Dis.* **99** 13-23.

Sakethoo K., Yergin B.M., Januskiewicz A., Kovitz K. and Sackner M.A. (1978) The effect of nasal decongestants on nasal mucus velocity. *Am. Rev. Resp. Dis.* **118** 251-254.

Sakakura Y., Ukai R., Matima Y., Murai S., Harada T. and Myoshi Y. (1983) Nasal mucociliary clearance under various conditions. *Acta Otolaryngol.* **96** 167-173.

Salzman R., Manson J.E., Griffing G.T., Kimmerle R., Ruderman N., McCall A., Stolz E.I., Mullin C., Small D., Armstrong J. and Melby J.C. (1985) Intranasal aerosolized insulin. Mixed-meal studies and long-term use in type 1 diabetes. *N. Engl. J. Med.* **312** 1078-1084.

Shionoiri H. and Kaneko Y. (1986) Intranasal administration of alpha-human natriuretic peptide produces a prolonged diuresis in healthy man. *Life Sciences* **38** 773-778.

Snow S.S., Logan T.P. and Hollender M.H. (1980) Nasal spray "addiction" and psychosis: a case report. *Br. J. Psychiat.* **136** 297-299.

Stanley P.J., Wilson R., Greenstone M.A., MacWilliam L. and Cole P.J. (1986) Effect of cigarette smoking on nasal mucociliary clearance and ciliary beat frequency. *Thorax* **41** 519-523.

Stuart B.O. (1973) Deposition of inhaled aerosols. *Arch. Int. Med.* **131** 60-73.

Su K.S.E., Campanale K.M., Mendelsohn L.G., Kerchner G.A. and Gries C.L. (1985) Nasal deliver of polypeptides, 1. Nasal absorption of enkephalins. *J. Pharm. Sci.* **74** 394-398.

Torjussen W. and Solberg A. (1976) Histological findings in the nasal mucosa of nickel workers. *Acta Otolaryngol.* **82** 132-134.

Van de Donk H.J.M. and Mercus F.W.H.M. (1981) Nasal drops: do they damage ciliary movement? *Pharmacy International* **2** 157.

Van de Donk H. J. M., Van Egmond A.L.M., Van den Huevel A.G.M., Zuidema J. and Mercus F.W.H.M. (1982) The effects of drugs on ciliary motility. I Decongestants. *Int. J. Pharmaceut.* **12** 57-65.

Vinther B. and Elbrond D. (1978) Nasal mucociliary function during penicillin treatment. *Acta Otolaryngol.* **86** 266-267.

Visor G.C., Bajka E. and Benjamin E. (1986) Intranasal absorption of Nicardipine in the rat. *J. Pharm. Sci.* **75** 44-46.

Wolfsdorf J., Swift D.L. and Avery M.E. (1969) Mist therapy reconsidered: an evaluation of the respiratory deposition of labelled water aerosols produced by jet and ultrasonic nebulizers. *Paediatrics* **43** 799-808.

10

Pulmonary Drug Delivery

Neena Washington, Clive G. Wilson and Clive Washington*
* Department of Pharmaceutical Sciences, Nottingham University,
University Park, Nottingham, NG7 2RD.

The major function of the pulmonary system is the oxygenation of blood and the removal of carbon dioxide. Breathing ventilates the respiratory tissue leading to gaseous exchange in the lungs. The tissue is therefore specialised to present the largest available surface area within the protection of the thorax. This is necessary to support the high metabolic rate of mammals.

The respiratory system in man is divided into the upper and lower respiratory tracts. The upper respiratory tract consists of the nose, nasal passages, paranasal passages, mouth, eustachian tubes, the pharynx, the oesophagus and the larynx. The trachea and bronchi are sometimes included as part of the upper respiratory tract. The lower respiratory tract consists of the true respiratory tissue, i.e. the air passages and alveoli.

Pulmonary drug delivery is primarily used to treat conditions of the respiratory tract although in recent years the possibility of systemic absorption of peptides and other molecules which are not absorbed through the gastrointestinal tract has been explored. Nebulisers, dry powder inhalers and metered dose inhalers are currently the most common devices used to deliver pharmaceutical preparations to the lung. The drugs delivered must be deposited onto the bronchial epithelium in therapeutic quantities but generally only about 10% of the dose delivered remains in the lungs (Newman *et al.*, 1982). The process is inefficient due to a combination of the mode of delivery, the point of inspiration relative to triggering the device and respiratory variables such as the breathing pattern. The anatomy and physical state of the respiratory tract can also markedly affect the inhalation, deposition, retention and activity of inhaled particles. Additionally, structures in the upper airways function to minimise the inhalation of particulate materials, and thus efficient delivery must overcome the ability of the lung to filter particles and remove them by mucociliary action (Ganderton and Jones, 1987).

STRUCTURE AND FUNCTION OF THE PULMONARY SYSTEM.
Upper Airway
As discussed in Chapter 9, the function of the nose is to provide humidification, filtration and warming of the inspired air. Although the nose is designed as the primary route of entry for gases, most people also breathe through the mouth particularly during stress and in this case many of the nasal defensive pathways are lost. Inhaled micro-organisms and dust are removed by sedimentation and impaction on to the mucus blanket which covers the respiratory epithelium.

Structure of the tracheo-bronchial tree
The tracheo-bronchial tree can be subdivided into the central airways (bronchi) and peripheral airways (bronchioles). In an adult, the trachea is 11 to 13 cm in length and 1.5 to 2.5 cm in diameter, and bifurcates to form the right and left main bronchi (Figure 10.1). The right bronchus divides into the upper, middle and lower branches

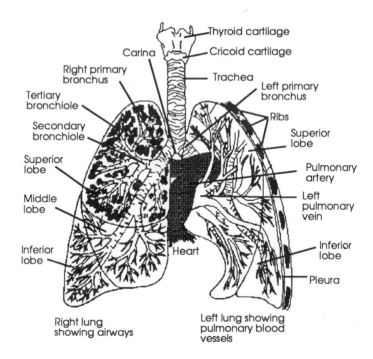

Figure 10.1. - Structure of the lungs

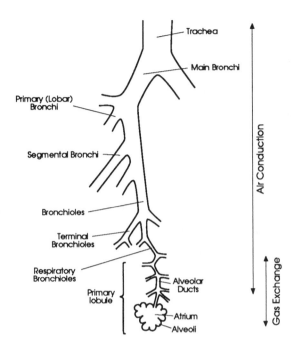

Figure 10.2. - The tracheo-bronchial tree

whilst the left bronchus divides only into an upper and a lower branch. These lobar bronchi give rise to branches called 'segmental bronchi'. The branching angle of 37° appears to be optimal to ensure smooth air flow.

Every branching of the tracheo-bronchial tree produces a new 'generation' of tubes, the total cross-sectional area increasing with each generation (Figure 10.2). The main bronchi are known as the first generation, the second and third generations are the lobar and segmental bronchi respectively. The fourth to ninth generations are the small bronchi and in these segmental bronchi the diameters decrease from approximately 4 to 1 mm. At a diameter of less than 1 mm they lie inside the lobules and are then correctly termed bronchioles. Here the function of the tissue changes from conducting airway to gas exchange. Although the decrease in diameter minimises the deadspace (the amount of gas not in contact with the respiratory surface), it is associated with a large increase in resistance to flow. A 10% reduction in diameter is associated with an increase in airway resistance of more than 50%. Thus, the airways should be as wide as possible to minimise resistance which, of course, increases deadspace. In the body these opposing factors are balanced by finely tuned physiological control which is easily disturbed by lung pathologies such as asthma and bronchitis.

The parenchyma of the lung, the region for gaseous exchange, consists of approximately 130,000 lobules each with a diameter of about 3.5 mm and containing around 2,200 alveoli. Each lobule is believed to be supplied by a single pulmonary arteriole. The terminal bronchioles branch into approximately 14 respiratory bronchioles, each of which branches further into the alveolar ducts. The ducts carry 3 or 4 spherical atria which lead to the alveolar sacs supplying 15-20 alveoli (Figure 10.3). Additional alveoli arise directly from the walls of the alveolar ducts, and these are responsible for approximately 35% of the total gas exchange. It has been estimated that there are 300 million alveoli in an adult human lung. The volume of an alveolus changes with the degree of inflation, but assuming 75% lung inflation,

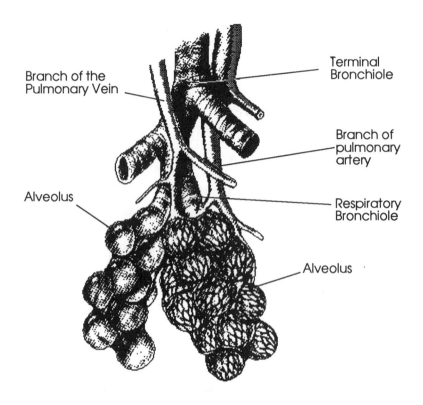

Figure 10.3. - Arrangement of alveoli

the diameter of an alveolus is thought to be between 250 and 290 μm. Weibel in 1963 estimated that each alveolus had a volume of 1.05×10^{-5} ml, with an air-tissue interface of 27×10^{-4} cm². For these calculations, it was assumed that the lung had a total air volume of 4.8 L, a total respiratory zone volume of 3.15 L and a total alveolar air-tissue interface of 81 m².

Epithelium
Upper Airways
The nasal cavity, the nasopharynx, larynx, trachea and bronchi are lined with pseudostratified, ciliated, columnar epithelium with many goblet cells. There are also coarse hairs in the nasal region of the respiratory tract.

Bronchi and Bronchioles
The bronchi, but not the bronchioles, have mucous and serous glands present. The bronchioles, however, possess goblet cells. The epithelium in the terminal and respiratory bronchioles consists largely of ciliated, cuboidal cells and smaller numbers of Clara cells. The ciliated epithelial cells each have about 20 cilia with an average length of 6 μm and a diameter of 0.3 μm. Each cilium is composed of a central doublet and 9 peripheral filaments which function as a structural support. Contractions result in successive beats of the cilia creating a wave which consists

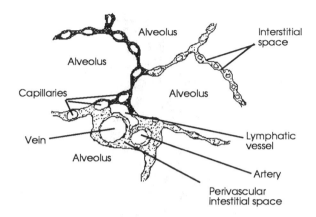

Figure 10.4. - Alveolar-capillary membrane

of a fast propulsion stroke followed by a slow recovery stroke. Clara cells become the most predominant cell type in the most distal part of the respiratory bronchioles. They have ultrastructural features of secretory cells but the nature and function of the secretory product is poorly understood.

Alveoli

In the alveolar ducts and alveoli the epithelium is flatter and becomes the simple, squamous type, 0.1 to 0.5 μm thick. The alveoli are packed tightly and do not have separate walls; adjacent alveoli being separated by a common alveolar septum with communication between alveoli via alveolar pores (Figure 10.4). The alveoli form a honeycomb of cells around the spiral, cylindrical surface of the alveolar duct (Figure 10.3). The exposed alveolar surface is normally covered with a surface film of lipoprotein material.

There are several types of pulmonary alveolar cells. Type I (or small type A), are non-phagocytic, membranous pneumocytes. These surface-lining epithelial cells are approximately 5 μm in thickness and possess thin squamous cytoplasmic extensions that originate from a central nucleated portion. These portions do not have any organelles and hence they are metabolically dependent on the central portion of the cell. This reduces their ability to repair themselves if damaged.

Attached to the basement membrane are the larger alveolar cells (Type II, type B or septal cells). These rounded, granular, epithelial pneumocytes are approximately 10 to 15 μm in thickness. There are 6 to 7 cells per alveolus and these cells possess great metabolic activity. They are believed to produce the surfactant material which lines the lung and to be essential for alveolar repair after damage from viruses or chemical agents.

Macrophages are also found in the lung. They are large, free mono-nuclear cells which contain lysosomes and they are found on the alveolar lining or in the free space. These phagocytic cells ingest exogenous and endogenous debris and are continually removed from the lung by the ciliary escalator, or move into the lymph nodes.

The remaining cell types include endothelial cells of the pulmonary blood capillaries, fibroblasts, histocytes and migratory blood cells.

Alveolar-Capillary Membrane

The blood and alveolar gases are separated by the alveolar capillary membrane (Figure 10.4) which is composed of a continuous epithelium of 0.1 to 0.5 μm thickness, a collagen fibre network, a ground substance, a basement membrane and the capillary endothelium. The interstitium is composed of a basement membrane of the endothelium a ground substance and epithelium. It forms a three dimensional skeleton to which the alveoli and capillaries are attached. Maximum absorption probably occurs in the areas where the interstitium is the thinnest (80 nm) since the surfactant is also thin in these areas (15 nm). Drainage of the interstitial fluid occurs by passage into the lymphatics, which often happens long after passage along the alveolar wall.

The thickness of the air-blood barrier varies from 0.2 μm to 10 μm (Weibel, 1969); although Divertie and Brown (1964) have reported values of between 0.4 to 2.1 μm depending upon the size of the intermembranous space. The barrier is minimal when the thickness is less than 0.5 μm since the epithelium and endothelium are present only as thin cytoplasmic extensions and the interstitium exists as a narrow gap between mostly fused membranes. When the diameter exceeds 0.5 μm additional structural elements are present. The minimal barrier thickness is nearly identical in structure and dimensions in all mammalian species that have been investigated (Weibel, 1969). This is in contrast to the alveolar surface areas which increase proportionally with body weight.

Lung Permeability

The alveolar epithelium and the capillary endothelium have a very high permeability to water, most gases and lipophilic substances. There is an effective barrier however for many hydrophilic substances of large molecular size and for ionic species. The alveolar type 1 cells have tight junctions, effectively limiting the penetration of molecules to those with a radius of less than 0.6 nm. Endothelial junctions are much larger, with gaps of the order of 4 to 6 nm. Clearance from the alveoli by passage across the epithelium bears an approximate inverse relationship to the molecular weight. The normal alveolar epithelium is almost totally impermeable to protein and small solutes, for example the half-time for turnover of albumin between plasma and the alveolar compartment is of the order of 36 hours (Straub, 1983). The microvascular endothelium, with its larger intercellular gaps, is far more permeable for all molecular sizes and there is normally an appreciable leak of protein into the systemic circulation.

Lung Mucus

A thin fluid layer called the mucous blanket, 5 μm in depth, covers the walls of the

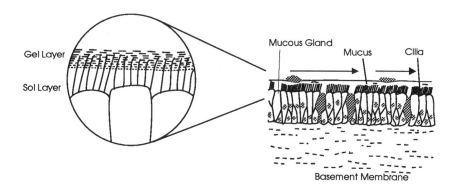

Figure 10.5. - Muco-ciliary escalator

entire respiratory tract (Figure 10.5). This barrier serves to trap foreign particles for subsequent removal and prevents dehydration of the surface epithelium by the unsaturated air taken in during inspiration.

There are about 6000 tracheo-bronchial glands in man, with an average of one cell per square millimetre of surface area. The ratio of goblet cells to ciliated cells is 1 to 5 in the large airways and 1 to several hundred in the bronchioles. The mucus largely originates from the vagally-innervated submucosal glands, with a smaller contribution from goblet cells. Within the gland, distal serous cells secrete a watery fluid, whereas the mucus cells near the neck secrete a gel. It is speculated that the secretions of the serous cells help in the movement of the swollen gel to the surface. Although the mucus producing cells are under vagal control and can be regulated by cholinergically mediated drugs, goblet cells discharge mucus without physiological stimulation.

The main component of nasal mucus appears to be a mucopolysaccharide complexed with sialic acid. Mucus contains 2-3% mucin, 1 to 2% electrolytes, and the remainder water. Tracheo-bronchial mucus has viscoelastic properties and it averages 5% solids, including 2% mucin, 1% carbohydrate, less than 1% lipid and 0.03% DNA. Pulmonary secretions are slightly hyperosmotic, but that secreted from the smaller bronchi and bronchioles are thought to be isosmotic, being in equilibrium with tissue and vascular fluids. The pH of rat tracheal secretions has been reported to be between 6.0 and 7.6.

Nasal mucus moves down, whereas tracheo-bronchial mucus moves upwards, to the hypopharynx at the rate of 2 cm min^{-1}. The mucus is then swallowed. A cross-section through the bronchial epithelium shows a mucous layer, cilia, serous fluid bathing the cilia, ciliated cells interspersed by mucus-secreting goblet cells, basal cells and a basement membrane (Figure 10.5). The mucus gel layer floats above the sol layer which has been calculated to be approximately 7 μm thick. The cilia extend through this layer so that the tip of the villus protrudes into the gel. This provides an efficient self-cleansing mechanism referred to as the muco-ciliary escalator. The co-ordinated movement of the cilia propels the mucous blanket and deposited foreign materials towards the pharynx where they are swallowed. It has been estimated that 1 litre of mucus is cleared every 24 hours. The composition of expectorated liquid and sputum varies, but consists of tracheo-bronchial, salivary, nasal and lacrimal gland secretions plus entrapped foreign material, dead tissue cells, phagocytes, leucocytes, alveolar lining and products of microbial infections.

Increased mucus secretion is brought about by cholinergic and α-adrenergic agonists which act directly on the mucus secreting cells of the submucosal gland. Serous secretions are stimulated by β-agonists or cholinergic stimulation whereas the goblet cells do not appear to be innervated. The peripheral granules in which the mucus is stored, are discharged continuously and form a reservoir which is secreted after exposure to an irritant stimulus (Neutra *et al*., 1984). Disease states can drastically change the distribution of goblet cells and composition of respiratory tract fluids. Conditions such as chronic bronchitis are characterised by increased sputum and chronic irritation leading to an increased number of glandular and goblet cells which result in a crowding of ciliated cells. Mucus transport is thus slowed and the problem is exacerbated by the increased viscosity of the mucus.

Lung Surfactant

The elastic fibres of the lung and the wall tension of the alveoli would cause the lung to collapse, if this were not counterbalanced by the presence of the lung surfactant system which covers the alveolar surface to the thickness of 10 to 20 nm. The surfactant has a liquid crystalline or gel structure which consists of phospholipids (74 %), mucopolysaccharides and possibly proteins. It forms a continuous covering over the alveoli and is constantly renewed from below. Fifty percent of the surfactant comprises of dipalmitoyl lecithin, replacement of which is rapid with a half-life of 14 hours. The surfactant can be destroyed by enzymes, lipids and detergents. If the surfactant is removed by irrigation of the lung with saline, no harm appears to result since it is rapidly replaced.

Blood Supply

The pulmonary artery arises from the right ventricle of the heart and thus supplies the lung with de-oxygenated blood. It receives a supply of oxygenated blood from the bronchial arteries. Smaller capillaries branch from the main arteries to supply the terminal bronchioles, respiratory bronchioles, alveolar ducts, air sacs and alveoli. The average internal diameter of the alveolar capillary is only 8 μm with an estimated total surface area of 60 to 80 square metres and a capillary blood volume of 100 to 200 ml. The large surface area allows rapid absorption and removal of any substance which may penetrate the alveoli-capillary membrane thereby producing good sink conditions for drug absorption. Blood takes only a few seconds to pass through the lungs and it has been estimated that the time for passage through the alveolar capillaries of males at rest to be 0.73 ± 0.3 s, falling to 0.34 ± 0.1 s on exercise.

Lymphatic System
In the adult lung, the lymphatic channels surround the bronchi, pulmonary arteries
and veins. A deep system of lymphatics lies adjacent to the alveoli. Movement of
fluid from the alveolar lumen to the lymphatics has been described as a two-stage
process. The first step is the passage across the epithelial lining through the
intercellular clefts and/or through the cytoplasmic layer by diffusion or pinocytosis.
The second step is the movement of fluid along the alveolar wall into the lymphatic
area.

Nervous Control
The tracheo-bronchial tree is supplied by both sympathetic and parasympathetic
nerves. The primary role of these nerves is the control of ventilation of the lungs
under varying physiological demand and also to protect the lung by the cough reflex,
bronchoconstriction and the secretion of mucus. The lung is heavily innervated, as
are the smooth muscle sheets which surround the airways, the intercostal muscles
and the diaphragm.

Stimulation of the sympathetic nerves via the β_2 adrenergic receptors primarily
results in active relaxation of bronchial smooth muscle. Stimulation of parasympathetic nerves via the nicotinic and muscarinic receptors results in increased
glandular activity and constriction of bronchial smooth muscle.

Cough Reflex
Cough receptors are found at the carina (the point at which the trachea divides into
the bronchi) and bifurcations of the larger bronchi. They are much more sensitive
to mechanical stimulation, and inhalation of dust produces bronchoconstriction at
low concentration and elicits the cough reflex with larger amounts (Widdicombe *et
al.*, 1962). Lung irritant receptors, located in the epithelial layers of the trachea and
larger airways, are much more sensitive to chemical stimulation and produce a
reflex bronchoconstriction and hyperpnoea (over respiration) on stimulation by
irritant gases or histamine given topically or by intravenous injection. The
constriction is relieved by isoprenaline or atropine which suggests that the effect is
due to contraction of smooth muscle, mediated through post-ganglionic cholinergic
pathways.

Biochemical Processes which occur in the Lung
Almost all of the drug-metabolizing enzymes found in the liver are also present in
the lung, although in much smaller amounts (Bend *et al.*, 1985). The lung has been
observed to be responsible for:
1) the removal and release of 5-hydroxytryptamine from the circulation
2) synthesis of prostaglandins
3) conversion of angiotensin I to the potent vasoconstrictor angiotensin II
4) release of histamine during certain pathological conditions and also uptake of
histamine from the venous blood followed by inactivation
5) inactivation of bradykinin which is involved in many allergic reactions in other
mammals, although it does not appear to have a similar involvement in humans.

The mast cells located around the small blood vessels and in the alveolar walls are rich in histamine, heparin, 5-hydroxytryptamine and hyaluronic acid. Histamine release accounts for many of the symptoms of bronchial asthma and allergies. It causes capillary dilatation, increased capillary permeability, contraction and spasm of smooth muscle, skin swelling, hypotension and increased secretion of saliva, mucus, tears and nasal fluids.

The mammalian lung can actively synthesize fatty acids, particularly palmitic and linoleic, and incorporate these into phospholipids which are predominantly saturated lecithins. The active synthesis of proteins by the alveolar cells has also been reported (Massaro, 1967).

FACTORS AFFECTING PARTICLE DEPOSITION IN THE LUNG

Lung function is directed towards preventing particles from entering, and clearing those that succeed, while drug delivery is directed towards overcoming this process. Aerosols used by patients should reach the desired location in sufficient quantity to be effective, and hence it is important to consider the factors which influence the amount and distribution of retained aerosols.

The physical characteristics of the aerosol cloud such as particle size, velocity, charge, density and hygroscopicity will affect its penetration and deposition. Deposition is also affected by physiological variables, including respiration rate, airway diameter, presence of excessive mucus and respiratory volume.

Physicochemical Properties

The three main mechanisms of deposition are inertial impaction, sedimentation and Brownian diffusion, the particle diameter determining the most important deposition mechanism (Figure 10.6).

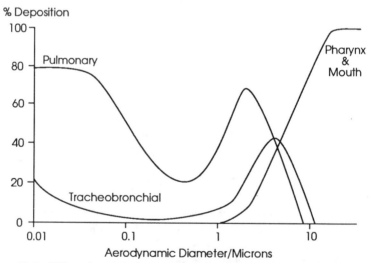

Figure 10.6. - Effect of particle size on deposition of a monodisperse aerosol (redrawn from Gonda, 1981)

Inertial impaction is the most important mechanism of deposition for particles greater than 5 μm in diameter (Raabe *et al.*, 1986). If particles are large or are travelling at high velocities they may be unable to follow a change in direction in the airstream, for example in the upper airways at bifurcations, and hence they will impact on the airway walls. Impacted deposition is also enhanced where airways are partially obstructed at high flow rates, and by a turbulent airflow in the trachea and major bronchi. Sedimentation occurs when particles settle under gravity. The rate of settling is proportional to the square of the particle diameter (Stokes' law) and so becomes less important for small particles. Brownian diffusion is an important mechanism of deposition only for particles less than about 0.5 μm in diameter. The particles are displaced by random bombardment of gas molecules and collide with airway walls.

As a consequence of physical forces acting on the droplet, the deposition of particulates in the lung is highly dependent on their diameter. Droplets larger than 10 μm impact in the upper airways and are rapidly removed by mucociliary processes. Smaller droplets which escape impaction in the upper airways, in the range 0.5 to 5 μm, are sufficiently large to deposit by sedimentation, while those below 0.5 μm are too small to sediment efficiently and migrate to the vessel walls by Brownian motion. The optimum diameter for pulmonary penetration has been determined by studies of the deposition of monodisperse aerosols (Gonda, 1981) and has been found to be 2 to 3 μm. Smaller particles are exhaled before sedimentation can occur, although breath-holding can improve deposition in these cases. Extremely small aerosols, below 0.1 μm, appear to deposit very efficiently through Brownian diffusion to the vessel walls, but such fine aerosols are extremely difficult to produce.

Often the particle size does not remain constant as an aerosol moves from the delivery system into the respiratory tract. Volatile aerosols may become smaller through evaporation whereas hygroscopic aerosols may grow dramatically. The exact relative humidity within airways is not known, but particles produced from dry atmospheric aerosols have been found to double in diameter when the relative humidity is increased to 98%. Moren and Andersson (1980), found that particle growth due to absorption of moisture did not appear to affect total drug deposition in the respiratory tract.

Air in the deep branches of the lung has been estimated to contain around 44 g water per cubic metre. An aerosol containing less moisture than 44 g m^{-3} will take up water from the mucosal surface when it is inhaled. Most aerosol particles will absorb moisture to a degree that depends on temperature, relative humidity and the nature of the aerosol particle. The degree of saturation is also device dependent since aerosols formed by jet nebulisers may have a very low humidity, while ultrasonic nebulisers produce an aerosol with a much higher humidity (Sara and Currie 1965; Graff and Benson 1969).

Thermophoresis of particles has been reported to occur in the lung. This is a movement of droplets towards the cooler areas due to the more rapid Brownian motion in the warm areas. It is thought that this effect is small and short-lived and the epithelial surface would repel the aerosol particles since the mucosa is generally warmer than the aerosol administered. Finally, electrostatic effects, in which the droplets are attracted to the vessel walls by virtue of a surface charge interaction, are thought to be unimportant in pulmonary delivery.

Physiological Variables
The average respiratory rate is approximately 15 breaths per minute with a tidal volume of about 500 ml and a residence time for tidal air of 3 seconds. A slowing of the respiratory rate increases the dwell time and retention of aerosol particles in the lung. Although increasing the respiratory rate decreases dwell time, it increases the turbulent flow and particle velocity. When flow becomes turbulent, the density rather than the viscosity affects the flow rate. Severe turbulence retards flow of gases into and out of the lung and results in premature deposition of the aerosol particles high into the respiratory tract since the collision rate with the walls is increased. Slowing inspiration and expiration minimises turbulent flow. Valberg and coworkers (1983) found by experimentation in dogs that total deposition decreased as breathing frequency increased; slow, deep breathing produced uniform deposition throughout the lung, but with little deposition in large airways; rapid, shallow ventilation resulted in enhanced large airway deposition, and slow, shallow breathing at high end-expiratory volumes enhanced small-airway deposition.

A highly significant change in the effective anatomy of the respiratory system occurs when there is a switch between nose and mouth breathing. In nose breathing, the combination of a small cross-section for airflow, sharp curves and interior nasal hairs helps to maximise particle impaction. Significant fractions of inhaled particles and droplets can be deposited in the nose and pharynx (Newman *et al.*, 1980).

The total pressure within the trachea is equal to atmospheric pressure, but during inspiration the pressure may drop to 60 to 100 mm Hg below atmospheric pressure, creating the gradient responsible for the inward flow of the aerosol cloud. The flow into each segment of the lung may vary considerably according to the pressure differential across each passageway and its resistance. Increasing the pressure differential increases the flow and penetration by aerosols. A popular method to increase the pressure differential is to use intermittent positive-pressure breathing.

Effects of Disease
The inhalation of aerosols, their penetration and deposition into the lungs, their absorption and activity is affected by the severity of pulmonary disease. The diseases are usually classified into the following major groups:
1) *Microbial infections* which can cause significant disturbances to respiratory physiology, such as increasing lung rigidity, a decrease in tidal volume and an increase in respiratory rate. Irritation, oedema and cough may also occur with an

increase in secretion and some degree of airway blockage.

2) *Pneumoconiosis* which is a disease characterised by lesions resulting from inhalation and retention of dust. This may result in fibrosis, mechanical obstruction of fine airways, oedema, local irritation and reflex bronchoconstriction.

3) *Carcinomas and tumors* causing airway obstruction.

4) *Obstructive lung disease* including atelectasis, bronchial asthma, chronic bronchitis and emphysema. These conditions may cause cough, increased mucus production, oedema, bronchoconstriction, plugging of the bronchioles and changes in pulmonary circulation, heart rate and blood pressure. The disease may lead to the destruction of alveolar ducts, sacs and respiratory bronchioles. In asthma, the bronchiole is more muscular which causes an invagination of the airway decreasing calibre. The increase in muscularity appears to be due to the presence of pro-inflammatory cells which establish a low level chronic hyper-responsiveness of pulmonary smooth muscle.

5) *Miscellaneous disease conditions* Acid-base disorders, e.g. acidosis, which causes hyperventilation and alkalosis which results in hypoventilation.

Respiratory diseases often affect the distribution of inspired particles. Bronchoconstriction or obstruction of airways will lead to diversion of flow to non obstructed airways. In advanced disease the remaining airways and alveoli may be increasingly exposed to inspired particles. Narrowing of airways by mucus, inflammation or bronchial constriction can increase linear velocities of airflow, enhance inertial deposition and cause more deposition in the central airways.

It has been demonstrated by Straub (1978) and Basran and coworkers (1985) that in adult respiratory distress syndrome, characterised by acute inflammatory oedema, the lung permeability to proteins increases and accumulation of fluid occurs.

Removal of Particles from the Alveoli

The major clearance mechanisms of inhaled particles include cough, sneeze, mucociliary transport and systemic absorption. Inhaled particles reaching the alveoli are removed by the alveolar phagocytes or "dust cells" since this region is not ciliated. These cells engulf the particulate and migrate to the ciliated areas of the bronchial tree, where they are transported up the muco-ciliary escalator. Some macrophages with engulfed particles slowly penetrate the alveolar wall, especially in the region of the alveolar duct, pass into the tissue fluid and lymphatics.

A study of technetium-99m labelled macroaggregated albumin aerosol (Tzila Zwas *et al.*, 1987) has demonstrated that after inhalation of the aerosol, radioactive boli were seen to move to the main bronchi after accumulating in regional lymph nodes and ascending towards the carina. The mean mucociliary clearance rate was 4.7 ± 1.3 mm min^{-1} in normal subjects and 8.2 ± 1.4 mm min^{-1} in bronchiectatic patients. Cigarette smokers demonstrate a considerable slowing in the clearance mechanisms of the large airways, resulting in an accumulation at the hilius, the junction between the lymph node and efferent lymphatic vessel (Sanchis *et al.*, 1970).

Assessment of Deposition

One of the most convenient methods to assess the pattern of distribution of therapeutic aerosols is by the use of imaging using a variety of radiopharmaceuticals. Diagnostically, these compounds are used to monitor lung ventilation as an alternative to using radioactive gases (Agnew *et al.*, 1982). Unfortunately, it is generally difficult to select radiopharmaceuticals which are suitable analogues of bronchodilators or corticosterioids. If the drug particles do not dissolve, such as those delivered from a dry powder inhaler, they can be labelled by co-precipitation or co-crystallization with a soluble label such as $^{99}Tc^m$pertechnetate (Vidgren *et al.*, 1987). A bronchodilator, the anti-cholinergic compound ipratropium bromide, has been labelled using a cyclotron-produced radionuclide ^{77}Br. This radionuclide has a half life of 58 hours with peak gamma-ray energies of 239 and 521 KeV which are not ideal but are usable for scintigraphic studies. The powder produced was incorporated into pressurised canisters and it was shown that upon actuation, radioactivity was lost from the canisters at a rate equal to that of the drug. The radiopharmaceutical was thus shown to be a valid marker of the distribution of the bronchodilator in the lungs (Short *et al.*, 1981). Malton (1984) used a tetraphenylarsonium complex to label salbutamol base which was then administered to dogs in a metered dose inhaler.

Deposition can also be followed using inert liquid droplets released from nebulisers or metered dose inhalers using technetium-99m labelled diethylenetriaminepentaaceticacid (DTPA) released from jet or ultrasonic nebulisers (Agnew *et al.*, 1982), or technetium-99m labelled phytate (Wasnich, 1976). Dolovich and coworkers (1981) used pertechnetate, fluorocarbon propellants and an ethanol co-solvent to make a pressurised aerosol formulation. Measurements of these soluble materials must be carried out immediately after inhalation since the tracers are absorbed rapidly via the lung. If a solution consisting of the drug substance and a radioactive material is nebulised, the droplets produced will contain both drug and radionuclide in proportions which will depend on their initial concentrations in the solutions. This technique is powerful since it can be used to measure both deposition of aerosol and clinical effect simultaneously in each volunteer. This technique was used to label oleic acid with iodine-131 in a salbutamol aerosol (Malton, 1984); however, it was found that the particle size distributions of drug and labelled compound differed, reducing the validity of the method.

The clearance from the lungs of smaller molecular weight species such as pertechnetate is more rapid than that of the larger molecules such as DTPA. This indicates that the rate of clearance depends upon the molecular size in relation to the size of the pores or the width of tight junctions between epithelial cells (Newman *et al.*, 1982). Materials such as $^{99}Tc^m$ stannous phytate show better alveolar deposition than pertechnetate or ^{111}In-DTPA with a slow clearance (Isitman *et al.*, 1974). It has been hypothesized that phytate bears a strong structural resemblance to triphosphoinositide, a component of the lung surfactant material, and that it binds to alveolar wall receptors competing for inositol receptors.

Krypton-81m gas is commonly used in diagnostic studies to show the total ventilated area of the lungs. This radioactive gas has a half-life of 13 seconds and therefore the subject is imaged while breathing in the gas. This method of assessing the ventilated area is useful since it is fairly quick to perform and the study results in a low radiation dose to the subject.

Conventional planar gamma scintigraphy does not allow clear distinction between central and peripheral deposition. Phipps and coworkers (1987) have used 3-dimensional gamma tomography to study the deposition of small and large droplets.

Drug Absorption
Inhaled drugs can be absorbed from their deposition site in various parts of the respiratory tract, including the upper airways, mouth, pharynx and lower airways. Each of these absorption sites may also be responsible for local metabolism of the drug. The drug reaching the lower airways may be metabolised in the bronchial wall and the lungs as well as being absorbed into the systemic circulation. Absorption from the gastrointestinal tract may also occur either due to direct swallowing of a portion of the aerosol, or from secondary swallowing following lung clearance. This can complicate measurements of absorption, but usually drugs which are effective when given orally are not administered as aerosols.

Lipid soluble drugs are usually absorbed by passive diffusion at rates that correlate with their lipid/water partition coefficients. Compounds which are poorly lipid-soluble are absorbed by diffusion through aqueous membrane pores, the absorption rate of the poorly lipid-soluble drugs being inversely related to their molecular size. Compounds such as disodium cromoglycate are at least partly absorbed by a saturable, carrier-type transport mechanism (Pauwels, 1982). Studies involving salbutamol administered from a pressurised aerosol (Walker *et al.*, 1972) showed that peak plasma levels were reached 3-5 hours after dosing, but the peak plasma level was probably related to the gastrointestinal absorption of the swallowed part of the aerosol dose. Another study involving terbutaline indicated that after inhalation, the peak plasma level was reached by 30 to 60 minutes (Nilson *et al.*, 1976). In this experiment ingested charcoal was used to prevent absorption from the gastrointestinal tract; without charcoal the peak plasma level was reached at 1-6 hours. This suggests that absorption from the airways is more rapid than from the gut. However, it may be possible that the peak plasma concentration results from absorption from the oral and pharyngeal mucosa.

The alveoli are a suitable area for drug absorption due to their large surface area and good blood supply. Taylor and coworkers (1965) calculated the permeability coefficient of several small lipid-insoluble substances across the alveolar-capillary membrane and concluded that the limiting portion of the barrier was the alveolar membrane itself. It is believed that this barrier exhibits passive transport character-istics similar to other organs lined with epithelial cells. The pulmonary capillary is more porous than the alveolar membrane, with a pore radius of 4 to 8 nm compared to 0.8 to 1.0 nm. Anaesthetics and respiratory gases are thought to cross the alveolar-capillary membrane quite readily, water crosses easily and in large quantities, but isotonic sodium chloride is only slowly absorbed. The membrane is only slightly permeable to aqueous solutes. Interestingly, high molecular weight amides and alkyl amines pass more readily than their low molecular weight homologues.

DRUGS ADMINISTERED VIA THE PULMONARY ROUTE

Drugs inhaled for the treatment of respiratory problems include sodium cromoglycate, a very powerful prophylactic drug used in the treatment of asthma. It has no direct bronchodilator action and it was formerly believed to act by preventing degranulation of mast cells and hence the release of histamine, but it now thought to have an additional actions such as inhibition of pulmonary sensory C-fibre discharge (Church, 1986; Richards et al., 1986). It is widely used in the management of extrinsic asthma and particularly exercise-induced asthma, and may also be effective in late onset asthma. The spinhaler is a common form of delivery system for this drug in powder form and recently cromoglycate has been formulated for administration by metered dose inhaler. Cromoglycate is also available for use in nebulisers as a solution, and is useful for children who have difficulty using a spinhaler or metered dose inhaler. A new drug in the category of anti-allergics is nedocromil sodium, which is equipotent with sodium cromoglycate (Riley et al., 1987).

Corticosteroids administered by inhalation are highly effective in controlling asthma with reduced systemic side-effects compared to an oral dose. They are used when other medication, e.g. ß-adrenoceptor agonists, has failed. Inhaled steroids have no direct bronchodilator effect, but they block late-onset asthmatic responses and may prevent or reverse airway hypersensitivity (Sotomayor et al., 1984; Fabbri et al., 1985). The drugs used, e.g. beclomethasone dipropionate, betamethasone and budesonide, exert a topical effect in the lungs but are inactivated when swallowed. The doses required are low (400 - 800 µg daily), resulting in low plasma concentrations thereby minimising systemic side effects. Modern treatment of asthma in childhood favours the use of small doses of steroid to keep inflammatory processes suppressed.

Beta adrenoceptor agonists including salbutamol, terbutaline and fenoterol are the most common type of drug given by metered dose inhaler as the standard first-line treatment in Britain for asthma and chronic obstructive airways disease. They provide rapid symptomatic relief where the predominant cause of reduced airway calibre is bronchial smooth muscle contraction, or they may be used as regular maintenance therapy to avert symptoms. Their preventative effect is particularly seen in the suppression of exercise-induced asthma (Clarke and Newman, 1984). Beta adrenoceptor agonists also increase the rate of mucociliary clearance, known to be abnormally slow in patients with obstructive airways disease. Inhaled ß-adrenoceptor agonists are less effective if airway inflammation is a major factor in the disease.

Other bronchodilators include anticholinergic drugs which act by blocking the muscarinic action of acetylcholine. A quaternary derivative of atropine, ipratropium bromide, is commonly delivered by nebuliser and has been successful in the control of acute asthma. Methyl-xanthines (theophylline and aminophylline) have been used for many years in the USA as a first line treatment for asthma. They are however less effective than ß-adrenoceptor agonists administered by aerosol (Clarke and Newman, 1984). Since reflex bronchoconstriction may be mediated through the stimulation of pulmonary sensory fibres, there is much interest in inhibition of this pathway as a future method of controlling asthma. Animal studies have demonstrated great potential for pulmonary delivery of suitable inhibitors which are currently being evaluated in man.

Various pharmacological agents alter the rheological function of mucus which has been exploited particularly to thin mucus to aid in its clearance from the bronchi. Water, saline and mucolytic aerosols are important as aids in the removal of the bronchial secretions which accumulate in chronic bronchitis, bronchiectasis, cystic fibrosis and asthma. Inorganic and organic iodides act directly on mucus and are used therapeutically. Addition of potassium iodide reduces the apparent viscosity (Martin *et al.*, 1980), presumably due to an effect of the halide on the configuration of the glycoprotein. Traditionally aerosols have been used in an attempt to liquefy secretions and induce sputum clearance, either by mucociliary action or coughing. Studies have shown that inhalation of water aerosol does liquefy and clear secretions (Palmer, 1960). It can however be an irritant and cause bronchoconstriction in asthmatics (Schoeffel *et al.*, 1981). Saline aerosol is bland and may well improve mucociliary clearance, particularly in a hypertonic concentration (7.1%) where it facilitates expectoration (Clarke and Newman, 1984). It may liquefy sputum by enhancing chloride (and water) flux across the bronchial mucosa (Nadel, 1981). Mucolytic aerosols are also widely used; N-acetyl-cysteine (Airbron) being best known in Britain, and 2 mercapto-ethane sulphonate (Mistabron) in Europe. Mistabron appears to enhance mucociliary clearance in patients with chronic bronchitis (Clarke *et al.*, 1979). Other molecules such as DL-penicillamine and dithiothreitol act on the sulphydryl bonds in mucus causing thinning, though nebulisation of dithiothreitol causes intense irritation and is therefore unsuitable for clinical exploitation (Lightowler and Lightowler, 1971).

On rare occasions antihistamines and antibiotics may by given as aerosols. Antibiotics are given because in asthmatics the mucus thickens and "plugs" the bronchiole. This plug may then become a focus for infection. Some antibiotics, notably the tetracyclines (Marriott and Kellaway, 1975), interact with mucus glycoprotein causing thickening. Mucus can also be thickened by addition of divalent and trivalent ions and the effect of copper ions is used as a method of controlling fertility, since if the mucus in the uterus is too thick, the sperm cannot penetrate through to the ovum. The exudates formed during inflammation and disease probably cause a mucus thickening by physical entrapment of mucus with biopolymers such as albumin, IgG, or IgA leading to changes in mucus viscoelasticity.

As has been mentioned, the pulmonary route has been used to achieve systemic delivery. A product containing ergotamine tartrate is available as an aerosolised dosage inhaler (360 µg per dose) which has the advantage of avoiding the delay in drug absorption due to gastric stasis associated with migraine. In vaccine delivery, aerosol administration of para-influenza Type 2 vaccine has been found to be more effective than subcutaneous injection (Wigley *et al.*, 1970). Penicillin reaches the bloodstream in therapeutic quantities after pulmonary delivery, but kanamycin is poorly absorbed from the lung and can be used for local drug delivery.

DOSAGE FORMS

Solutions must be converted into aerosols prior to administration to the lung. An aerosol consists of finely-divided liquid droplets or solid particles in a gaseous suspension. An atomiser is the general term for a device which generates an aerosol and may be electrically, pneumatically or mechanically powered. Pressurised inhalation aerosols are self-contained products which contain sufficient internal pressure to eject the material in the form of a spray. The active ingredient is usually dissolved in a liquefied propellant system with the aid of a co-solvent, or suspended in a micronised form using a surfactant. The two main types of device used at present to produce aerosols are nebulisers and metered dose inhalers.

Nebulisers

Nebulisers produce mists or clouds which are condensations of liquid droplets around nuclei suspended in a gas. Medical nebulisers can be divided into two main groups, pneumatic and electric. A pneumatic generator operates from a pressurised gas source, while an electric generator derives its power from an electric source. There are two types of pneumatic nebulisers (jet and hydrodynamic) and one electric generator (ultrasonic) presently used for medical purposes.

The jet nebuliser is a system in which a high-velocity gas flow is directed over a tube that is immersed in a water reservoir (Figure 10.7). The expansion of the driver gas

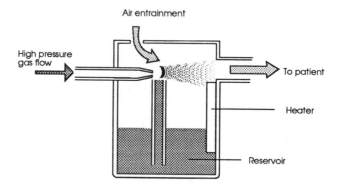

Figure 10.7. - Jet nebuliser

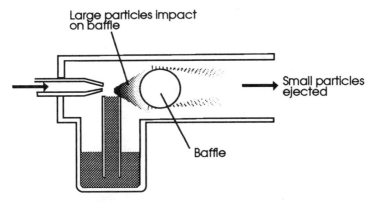

Figure 10.8. - Effect of a baffle on aerosol particle size

decreases the pressure over the tube, which draws the formulation into the gas stream. The high shear rate in the jet stream then nebulises it. The gross particles are then baffled into relatively uniform particle sizes. The gas pressure is supplied by a gas cylinder or compressor. A baffle is a device that deflects gas flow (Figure 10.8). When such a device is placed in the path of a gas flow that contains water particles, the large particles impact on the baffle and are deposited, while the smaller particles are deflected by the airstream as it moves around the baffle. The diameter of the emerging particles is normally in the range of 1-7 µm, depending on the gas pressure, and variables such as surface tension and viscosity.

The hydrodynamic nebuliser uses a system that prepares a film of water for aerosol formation by flowing it over a hollow sphere. A small orifice in the sphere expels gas at supersonic velocity. This high-velocity gas ruptures the thin film of water and produces a continuous dispersion of fine, liquid particles.

The ultrasonic nebuliser consists of a piezo-electric crystal which produces high frequency sound waves in the liquid in the nebulising unit. The surface waves produce small droplets (Faraday crispations) which are conducted away by an airstream for inhalation. The droplet diameters produced by the device depend on the ultrasonic driving frequency and the liquid properties, but are usually in the range 4-10 µm.

Generally, aqueous solvents are used in nebulisers, but organic solvents such as glycerin or propylene glycol may also be added. Polypropylene glycol is used in many aerosol formulations, but due to its hygroscopicity, solutions containing more than 95% w/v are deposited mainly in the upper respiratory tract. Stabilised aerosol droplets containing glycols have high surface tensions that cause them to rebound from the surfaces instead of depositing on them. Addition of a detergent increases aerosol deposition, presumably by decreasing the energy required to spread the droplet on the epithelial surface. Delivery of small quantities of solution to the lung generally does not require the formulation to be buffered or the tonicity to be controlled since the large surface area and dilution by the fluid lining of the lung make this unnecessary.

Pressurised Inhalation Aerosols

Usually the drug is a polar solid which has been dissolved or suspended in a non-polar liquified propellant. If the preparation is a suspension, the powder is normally micronised by fluid energy milling and wetted by the addition of a surfactant. Lecithin, oleic acid, and the Span and Tween series surfactants have been widely used for this type of formulation. Most drugs are poorly soluble in the chlorofluoro-carbons (CFCs) used as aerosol propellants, and hence co-solvents such as lower alkanols are used, e.g. ethanol or isopropanol, and usually there is a little water present. Mineral oils should be excluded from all sprays because of their potential to cause oil aspiration (lipoid) pneumonia. The selection of a propellant depends on a variety of factors such as miscibility with cosolvent and drug, vapour pressure, stability, and more recently environmental acceptability. Several manufacturers are considering the replacement of CFC propellants with materials such as dimethyl ether, despite the relatively small quantities of material involved.

Metered dose inhalers are the most commonly used drug delivery system for inhalation. They contain suspensions of fine drug particles or drug solutions in chlorofluorocarbon propellants. The propellants have a high vapour pressure of around 400 kPa at room temperature, but since the device is sealed, only a small fraction of the propellant exists as a gas. The canister consists of a metering valve crimped on to an aluminum can. Individual doses are measured volumetrically by a metering chamber within the valve. It is the latent heat of evaporation of the volatile propellants which provides the energy for atomisation.

The valve stem is fitted into an actuator incorporating a mouthpiece (Figure 10.9). The aerosol, consisting of propellant droplets containing drug, is delivered from the actuator mouthpiece at very high velocity, probably about 30 ms⁻¹ (Malton, 1984).

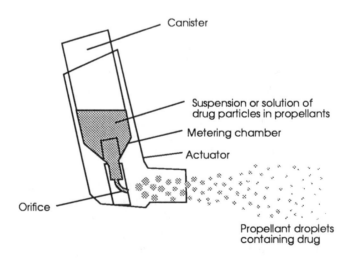

Figure 10.9. - Metered dose inhaler

There is partial (15 - 20%) evaporation of propellant prior to exit from the atomising nozzle, ("flashing") and further breakup of droplets beyond this point caused by the violent evaporation of the propellant. This results in a wide droplet size distribution from 1-5 μm. It has been found however, that only 10% of particulates delivered in a single dose released by a metered-dose inhaler actually reaches the lungs (Newman *et al.*, 1982), since the bulk of it impacts in the oropharynx and the mouthpiece. Recent studies conducted in our laboratories using $^{99}Tc^{m}$- hexamethylpropylamine oxine (HMPAO) delivered with a metered dose inhaler have shown that if the drug is soluble in propellant, as much as 26% of the dose can be absorbed into the lungs (Ashworth *et al.*, 1989).

In order to be effective, metered dose aerosols must be triggered as the patient is inhaling. Some patients have difficulty with this feat of coordination, and the Autohaler® has been designed to overcome this by triggering the valve as the patient breathes in.

Aerosol Powder Devices

For ease of use, powders intended for administration via the pulmonary route are often packaged in vials or capsules. The most commonly used excipient is lactose which acts as a diluent for the drug. The drug is usually micronised, but the diluent may have a larger particle size enabling it to be deposited in the upper respiratory tract, while the active agent can penetrate further into the lung.

There are several methods for delivering powders to the lung:
a) *The Aerohaler* (Abbott Laboratories, U.S.A.). This is a curved plastic tubular device, which is loaded with a sifter cartridge containing finely powdered formulation. The airstream produced by the patient inhaling causes a metal ball to strike the sifter cartridge, this shaking out a small amount of powder into the airstream.
b) *The Spinhaler* (Fisons Limited U.K.) This is a tubular plastic device which is loaded with a gelatin capsule containing drug powder. The capsule is pierced by two pins and when the patient inhales through the device, a rotor spins the capsule with an eccentric movement. The powder from the capsule is thrown into the airstream (Bell *et al.*, 1971). Unfortunately, up to 50% of the capsule dose is lost by deposition in the mouth and the back of the throat (Moss *et al.*, 1971). Vidgren and coworkers (1987) demonstrated by gamma scintigraphy that a typical dry powder formulation of sodium cromoglycate suffers losses of 44% in the mouth and 40% in the actuator nozzle itself.

CONCLUSIONS

The pulmonary route has received little attention as a potential route of entry for systemically acting compounds which are unstable in or poorly absorbed from the gastrointestinal tract. In the therapy of asthma where prophylactic treatment is an obvious advantage, there is a place for sustained release pulmonary dosage forms, if they can be employed. There has been some research on the delivery of sodium cromoglycate in liposomal preparations, which sustains high concentrations of drug in the lung (Taylor *et al.,* 1989), but generally the impetus has been slow. The worldwide movement to reduce the use of chlorofluorocarbon propellants will probably force innovation in aerosol delivery systems and perhaps controlled delivery through the pulmonary route will become possible.

REFERENCES

Agnew J.E., Francis R.A., Pavia D. and Clarke S.W. (1982) Quantitative comparison of $^{99}Tc^m$-aerosol and $^{81}Kr^m$ ventilation images. *Clin. Phys. Physiol. Meas.* **3** 21-30.

Ashworth H.L., Wilson C.G., Sims E.E., Wotton P. and Hardy J.G. (1989) Delivery of a propellant soluble drug from a metered dose inhaler. *in preparation*

Basran G.S., Byrne A.J. and Hardy J.G. (1985) A non-invasive technique for monitoring lung vascular permeability in man. *Nucl. Med. Commun.* **3** 3-10.

Bell J.H., Hartley P.S. and Cox J.S.G. (1971) Dry powder aerosols. 1. New powder inhalation device. *J. Pharm. Sci.* **60** 1559-1607.

Bend J.R., Serabjit-Singh C.J. and Philpot R.M. (1985) The pulmonary uptake, accumulation and metabolism of xenobiotics. *Ann. Rev. Pharmacol. Toxicol.* **25** 97-125.

Clarke S.W., Lopez-Vidriero M.T., Pavia D. and Thomson M.L. (1979) The effect of sodium-2-mercaptoethane sulphonate and hypertonic saline aerosols on bronchial clearance in chronic bronchitis. *Br. J. Clin. Pharmacol.* **7** 39-44.

Clarke S.W. and Newman S.P. (1984) Therapeutic aerosols 2- Drugs available by the inhaled route. *Thorax* **39** 1-7.

Church M.K. (1986) Is inhibition of mast cell mediator release relevant to the clinical activity of anti-allergenic drugs? *Agents and Actions* **18** 288-293.

Divertie M. and Brown A.L. (1964) The fine structure of the normal human alveolocapillary membrane. *JAMA* **187** 938-941.

Dolovich M.B., Ruffin R.E., Roberts R. and Newhouse M.T. (1981) Optimum drug delivery of aerosols from metered dose inhalers. *Chest* **80** 911-915.

Fabbri L.M., Chioesura-Corona P., Dal Vecchio L., di-Guiacomo G.R., Zocca E., de Marzo N., Mastrelli P. and Mapp C.E. (1985) Prednisone inhibits late asthmatic reactions and the associated increase in airway responsiveness induced by toluene-diisocyanate in sensitised subjects. *Am. Rev. Resp. Dis.* **132** 1016-1014.

Ganderton D. and Jones T.M. (1987) Introduction. In *"Drug Delivery to the Respiratory Tract"*. Ed Ganderton D. and Jones T.M., Chapter 1 Ellis Horwood Ltd., Chicester.pp9-12.

Gonda I. (1981) A semi-empirical model of aerosol deposition in the human respiratory tract for mouth inhalation. *J. Pharm. Pharmacol.* **33** 692-696.

Graff T.D. and Benson D.W. (1969) Systemic and pulmonary changes with inhaled humid atmospheres : clinical application. *Anaesthesiology* **30** 199-207.

Isitman A.T., Manoli R., Schmidt G.H. and Holmes R.A. (1974) An assessment of alveolar deposition and pulmonary clearance of radiopharmaceuticals after nebulisation. *Am. J. Roentgenol. Radium Ther. Nucl. Med.* **120** 776-781.

Lightowler J.E. and Lightowler N.M. (1971) Comparative mucolytic studies on dithiothreitol, N-acetylcysteine and L-cysteine on human respiratory mucus in vitro and their effects on the role of flow of mucus in the exposed trachea of the rat on topical administration. *Arch. Int. Pharmacodyn. Ther.* **189** 53-58.

Malton C.A. (1984) Deposition of Aerosols. Ph.D. Thesis, University of Nottingham.

Marriott C. and Kellaway I.W. (1975) The effect of tetracyclines on the viscoelastic properties of bronchial mucus. *Biorheology* **12** 391-395.

Martin R., Litt M. and Marriott C. (1980) The effect of mucolytic agents on the rheological and transport properties of canine tracheal mucus. *Am. Rev. Resp. Dis.* **121** 495-500.

Massaro D. (1967) Synthesis of proteins by alveolar cells. *Nature (London)* **215** 646-647.

Moren F. and Andersson J. (1980) Fraction of dose exhaled after administration of pressurised inhalation aerosols. *Int. J. Pharmaceut.* **6** 295-300.

Moss G.F., Jones K.M., Ritchie J.T. and Cox J.S.G. (1971) Plasma levels and urinary excretion of disodium cromoglycate after inhalation by human volunteers. *Toxicol. Appl. Pharmacol.* **20** 147-156.

Nadel J.A. (1981) New approaches on regulation of fluid secretions in airways. *Chest* **80** 849-851.

Neutra M.R., Phillips T.L. and Phillips T.E. (1984) In *Mucus and Mucosa*. Ciba Foundation Symposium no 109. Pitman London pp20.

Newman S.P., Pavia D. and Clarke S.W. (1980) Simple instructions for using pressurized aerosol bronchodilators. *J. Royal Soc. Med.* **73** 776-779.

Newman S.P., Agnew J.E., Pavia D. and Clarke S.W. (1982) Inhaled aerosols: lung deposition and clinical application. *Clin. Phys. Physiol. Meas.* **3** 1-20.

Nilson H.T., Simonsson B.G. and Strom B. (1976) The fate of ^{3}H-terbutaline sulphate administered to man as an aerosol. *Eur. J. Clin. Pharmacol.* **10** 1-7.

Palmer K.N.V. (1960) Reduction of sputum viscosity by a water aerosol in bronchitis. *Lancet* **1** 91.

Pauwels R. (1982) Pharmacokinetics of inhaled drugs. In "*Aerosols in Medicine. Principles, diagnosis and therapy*" Elsevier, Biomedical Sciences Division.

Phipps P.R., Gonda I., Bailey D.L., Borham P., Bautovich G. and Anderson S.D. (1987) Comparison of methods for the measurement of regional aerosol deposition. *J. Pharm. Pharmacol.* **39** 78P

Raabe O.G., Howard R.S. and Cross C.E. (1986) In *Bronchial Asthma*. Ed. Gershwin M.E., Grune and Stratton, London and New York. pp 495-514

Richards I.M., Dixon M., Jackson D.M. and Vendy K. (1986) Alternative modes of action of sodium cromoglycate. *Agents and Actions.* **18** 294-300.

Riley P.A., Mather M.E., Keogh R.W. and Eady R.P. (1987) Activity of neocromil sodium in mast cell dependent reactions in the rat. *Int. Arch. Allergy Appl. Immunol.* **82** 108-110.

Sanchis J., Dolovich M., Chalmers R. and Newhouse M.T. (1970) Regional distribution and lung clearance mechanisms in smokers and non-smokers. *Inhaled Particles and Vapours* **3** 183-191.

Sara C. and Currie T. (1965) Humidification by nebulisation. *Med. J. Aust.* **1** 174-179.

Schoeffel R.E., Anderson S.A. and Altounyan R.E.C. (1981) Bronchial hyper-reactivity in response to inhalation of ultrasonically nebulised solutions of distilled water and saline. *Br. Med. J.* **283** 1285-1287.

Short M.D., Singh C.A., Few J.D., Studdy P.T., Heaf P.J.D. and Spiro S.G. (1981) The labelling and monitoring of an inhaled, synthetic, anticholinergic bronchodilating agent. *Chest* **80** 918-921.

Sotomayer H., Badier M., Veruloet D. and Orehek J. (1984) Seasonal increase of carbachol airway responsiveness in patients allergic to grass pollen. Reversal by corticosteroids. *Am. Rev. Resp. Dis.* **130** 56-58.

Straub N.C. (1978) Pulmonary edema due to increased microvascular permeability to fluid and protein. *Circ Res.* **43** 143-151.

Taylor A.E., Guyton A.C. and Bishop V.S. (1965) Permeability of the alveolar membrane to solutes. *Circ. Res.* **16** 352-362.

Taylor K.M.G., Taylor G., Kellaway I.W. and Stevens J. (1989) The influence of liposomal encapsulation on sodium cromoglycate pharmacokinetics in man. *Pharm. Res.* **6** 633-636.

Tzila Zwas S., Katz I., Belfer B., Baum G.L. and Aharonson E. (1987) Scintigraphic monitoring of mucociliary tracheo-bronchial clearance of technetium-99m macroaggregated albumin aerosol. *J. Nucl. Med.* **28** 161-167.

Valberg P.A., Brain J.D., Sneddon S.L. and LeMott S.R. (1983) Breathing patterns influence aerosol deposition sites in excised dog lungs. *J. Appl. Physiol.* **53** 824-839.

Vidgren M.T., Kärkkäinen A., Paronen T.P. and Karjalainen P. (1987) Respiratory tract deposition of ^{99m}Tc-labelled drug particles administered via a drug powder inhaler. *Int. J. Pharmaceut.* **39** 101-105.

Walker S.R., Evans M.E., Richards A.J. and Paterson J.W. (1972) The clinical pharmacology of oral and inhaled salbutamol. *Clin. Pharmacol. Ther.* **13** 861-867.

Wasnich R.D. (1976) A high frequency ultrasonic nebuliser system for radioaerosol delivery. *J. Nucl. Med.* **17** 707-710.

Weibel E.R. (1963) Morphology of the human lung. Academic Press, New York.

Weibel E.R. (1969) Morphometric estimation of pulmonary diffusion capacity. 1. Model and methods. *Resp. Physiol.* **11** 54-75.

Widdicombe J.G., Kent D.C. and Nadel J.A. (1962) Mechanism of bronchoconstriction during inhalation of dust. *J. Appl. Physiol.* **17** 613-616.

Wigley F.M., Fruchtman M.H. and Waldman R.H. (1970) Aerosol immunisation of humans with inactivated parainfluenza type 2 vaccine. *N. Engl. J. Med.* **283** 1250-1253.

Index